AF869085

THE FATTY LIVER FIX

A Complete Guide to Understanding and Reversing Fatty Liver Disease Naturally

SACHA LUCAS

MagletPublishing

© Copyright Maglet Publishing 2024 - All rights reserved.

The content contained within this book may not be reproduced, duplicated or transmitted without direct written permission from the author or the publisher.

Under no circumstances will any blame or legal responsibility be held against the publisher, or author, for any damages, reparation, or monetary loss due to the information contained within this book, either directly or indirectly.

Legal Notice:

This book is copyright protected. It is only for personal use. You cannot amend, distribute, sell, use, quote or paraphrase any part, or the content within this book, without the consent of the author or publisher.

Disclaimer Notice:

Please note the information contained within this document is for educational and entertainment purposes only. All effort has been executed to present accurate, up to date, reliable, complete information. No warranties of any kind are declared or implied. Readers acknowledge that the author is not engaged in the rendering of legal, financial, medical or professional advice. The content within this book has been derived from various sources. Please consult a licensed professional before attempting any techniques outlined in this book.

By reading this document, the reader agrees that under no circumstances is the author responsible for any losses, direct or indirect, that are incurred as a result of the use of the information contained within this document, including, but not limited to, errors, omissions, or inaccuracies.

ISBN: 978-1-9167681-0-9

Contents

Introduction

Welcome to *The Fatty Liver Fix*, your comprehensive guide to understanding and reversing fatty liver disease through natural methods. Whether you're just learning about fatty liver disease or have been managing it for some time, this book is here to provide you with practical tools, insights, and encouragement to help you. We'll explore how you can make meaningful changes in your life to support your liver's health and, more importantly, how to sustain those changes long-term.

Fatty liver disease—particularly non-alcoholic fatty liver disease (NAFLD), is becoming increasingly common. It occurs when excess fat builds up in the liver, often due to poor diet, lack of exercise, or certain health conditions like obesity and diabetes. While it may sound scary, the good news is that, in many cases, fatty liver disease is reversible. With the right steps, you can take control of your liver health and work toward a healthier future.

But here's where it can feel overwhelming—where do you even begin? There's a lot of information out there, some of it helpful, some of it confusing, and it's easy to feel lost. That's where *The Fatty Liver Fix* comes in. We're here to cut through the noise and provide clear, simple steps that anyone can follow. We'll focus on natural approaches, which means no expensive treatments or miracle cures—just practical lifestyle changes you can start making today.

In this book, you'll learn how diet, exercise, stress management, and regular check-ups can have a huge impact on reversing fatty liver. These aren't one-size-fits-all solutions; instead, they're strategies that you can personalize based on your unique needs. You'll also find that the journey toward a healthier liver isn't just about your liver. It's about embracing a new mindset of overall wellness—one that can improve your energy, mood, and quality of life.

Throughout this book, we'll also cover some common myths about fatty liver disease, helping you separate fact from fiction. You'll understand the key role that your liver plays in your body and why it's so important to give it the care it deserves. We'll dive into easy, actionable tips for adjusting your diet, including foods that support liver health, and practical ways to increase your daily activity without feeling overwhelmed. You'll also learn about the connection between stress and liver health, along with simple mindfulness practices that can make a big difference in how you feel.

We'll explore real-life success stories from people who have reversed their fatty liver disease through natural methods, showing that it's possible to turn things around with dedication and the right knowledge. Most importantly, this book will empower you to take charge of your health journey, one step at a time.

So, whether you've just been diagnosed or have been managing your condition for a while, *The Fatty Liver Fix* is your guide to better health. Together, we'll explore how small, manageable changes can make a big difference. You're not alone in this journey, and with the right information and support, you can reclaim your health and feel your best again. Let's get started!

1

Fatty Liver Disease Explained

Your liver is an unsung hero. While it might not get as much recognition as your heart or brain, its role in maintaining your health is absolutely vital. Whether you've been recently diagnosed with fatty liver disease or simply want to understand more about this powerhouse organ, you've come to the right place.

Fatty liver disease, though common, can be confusing. There are myths, misunderstandings, and fears surrounding it, but knowledge is the first step in taking control of your health.

In this chapter, we'll strip away the mystery, starting with a deeper dive into the liver itself, what it does, how it works, and why it's so important. Once you truly understand your liver, managing and even reversing fatty liver becomes a much more achievable goal.

Let's begin by exploring the wonders of your liver and why keeping it healthy is essential for your overall well-being.

Why Your Liver Matters

The liver is one of the most hardworking organs in your body, responsible for performing over 500 vital functions every single day (Newman, 2018). Let's have a detailed look at some of these essential functions:

The Liver's Role in Filtering Toxins

Think of your liver as a skilled filter, working around the clock to keep your blood clean and free from harmful substances. Every time you eat, drink, or breathe in pollutants, your liver jumps in to process and remove toxins from your bloodstream. It breaks down everything from alcohol to environmental chemicals, making sure they don't pile up in your body and cause harm.

For instance, if you enjoy a glass of wine now and then, your liver is the one breaking down the alcohol into less harmful substances. Then, those substances are excreted through your kidneys or intestines. Without this detox process, everyday activities can overwhelm your body with toxins.

But the liver doesn't just filter; it also stores nutrients, like vitamins and minerals, and releases them into your bloodstream as needed. This balance is key to keeping your body functioning well (Newman, 2018).

You can picture the liver as a smart filter in your home. It doesn't just catch debris; it actively decides what should stay, what should go, and when something needs to be released. When your liver is working great, it can handle toxins efficiently. But if fatty liver disease sets in, the liver gets overwhelmed, making it tough to filter and detoxify. Over time, this can lead to inflammation and scarring, which makes it even harder for the liver to do its job right.

How Your Liver Supports Your Body

Beyond its role as a filter, your liver is a multitasking marvel when it comes to digestion and energy management. After you eat a meal, the liver plays an integral role in processing the nutrients you've consumed, especially fats, carbohydrates, and proteins.

- **Digestion and bile production:** One of the liver's key digestive functions is producing bile, a yellow-green fluid that helps break down fats into smaller, absorbable molecules. The bile is stored in the gallbladder and released into your small intestine during digestion. Without enough bile, fats would pass through your system without being properly digested, which can lead to digestive issues (Newman, 2018).
- **Energy storage and release:** After you eat, your liver also acts as a storage unit for glucose, a sugar that provides your body with energy. It stores glucose in the form of glycogen, which can be released back into your bloodstream when your body needs a quick burst of energy, such as between meals or during exercise. This function is especially important in maintaining stable blood sugar levels. When your liver becomes overloaded with fat, it can disrupt this process, creating imbalances in blood sugar, which can eventually result in conditions like type 2 diabetes (Newman, 2018).
- **Regulation of blood components:** Your liver also plays a huge role in regulating various components of your blood. It helps produce important proteins, such as albumin, which keeps fluids in your bloodstream from leaking into other tissues. The liver also produces clotting factors that

help prevent excessive bleeding when you're injured. Additionally, it breaks down old or damaged blood cells, recycling their components or sending them off for excretion.

The liver's capability to carry out these tasks depends on its overall health. When fatty liver disease begins to interfere, the liver's efficiency in digestion, energy storage, and blood regulation is affected. So, different metabolic and digestive problems are expected. For example, people with this liver condition often experience fatigue, which can be linked to the liver's reduced ability to manage glucose or handle nutrient absorption.

The Liver's Remarkable Ability to Heal

One of the coolest things about the liver is its ability to regenerate. Unlike many organs, the liver can repair itself, even after serious damage. This regenerative capability gives hope to many people with fatty liver. If you take the right steps, like improving your diet, exercising, and cutting back on alcohol, you can support your liver's healing process.

A great example of the liver's healing power comes from people who have partial liver transplants. In these cases, part of the liver is removed for donation or treatment. In a healthy person, the remaining liver can grow back to full size in just a few months, with minimal loss of function.

However, this resilience has limits. If this liver ailment goes untreated, the fat buildup can cause inflammation and lead to liver scarring (fibrosis) and eventually irreversible damage (cirrhosis). At that point, the liver's ability to regenerate goes way down, and the risk of serious complications like liver failure or cancer goes up (Newman, 2018).

The main goal is that fatty liver disease doesn't have to be a life sentence. Your liver is forgiving, especially if you catch problems early and make the right lifestyle changes.

What is Fatty Liver Disease?

Let's take a closer look at this condition. While it may seem daunting, gaining a better understanding empowers you to take control and take action. In this section, we'll break down the terminology around fatty liver disease, look at how common it is, and discuss the hopeful reality that early-stage fatty liver disease can often be reversed with lifestyle changes.

Breaking Down Fatty Liver Terms

Fatty liver disease is a term that encloses various conditions marked by an excessive accumulation of fat in the liver. While this may seem straightforward, the terminology can be confusing. Let's break it down:

- **Fatty Liver Disease (FLD)** is the overarching term that refers to any condition where fat builds up in the liver. It can be classified into two main categories: alcoholic and non-alcoholic fatty liver disease.
- **Non-Alcoholic Fatty Liver Disease (NAFLD)** is a specific type of FLD that occurs in people who drink little to no alcohol. It has gained attention as a significant health issue, particularly in the context of rising obesity rates and lifestyle-related diseases. NAFLD is marked by fat accumulation in the liver without inflammation or liver cell damage, making it the more benign of the two conditions (Newman, 2018).
- **Non-alcoholic steatohepatitis (NASH)** represents a more severe form of NAFLD, where fat

buildup is accompanied by liver inflammation and damage. This condition can lead to fibrosis (scarring of the liver) and even cirrhosis if not addressed. It's important to note that while NASH is part of the NAFLD spectrum, not everyone with NAFLD will progress to NASH (Newman, 2018).

Understanding these distinctions is fundamental for grasping the implications of fatty liver disease. While NAFLD may not present immediate health concerns, it can pave the way for more severe conditions if left unchecked.

How Common is Fatty Liver Disease

The prevalence of fatty liver is on the rise, and it's becoming a global health concern. Recent estimates suggest that NAFLD affects approximately 25-32% of adults worldwide, with numbers rising in both developed and developing countries (Newman, 2018).

In the United States, studies show that about one in four adults may have NAFLD, while 3-12% may progress to NASH (Newman, 2018). This growing epidemic can be attributed to various factors, including rising obesity rates, sedentary lifestyles, and poor dietary choices. For instance, a diet high in sugar, unhealthy fats, and processed foods can contribute to the development of fatty liver.

Certain demographics are more susceptible to developing NAFLD and NASH. For example, people with obesity, type 2 diabetes, high cholesterol, and metabolic syndrome are at a higher risk (Newman, 2018). Did you know that ethnicity also plays a role?

Yes, studies reveal that Hispanic people are more likely to

develop fatty liver disease compared to their Caucasian and African American counterparts (Rich et al., 2018).

The increasing diagnosis rate of fatty liver disorder is concerning, particularly since many people remain unaware they have it. The condition is often asymptomatic in its early stages, making regular health check-ups crucial for early detection. As healthcare providers become more aware of the prevalence of fatty liver sickness, there's a greater emphasis on screening for it during routine check-ups, especially in at-risk populations.

Can Fatty Liver Be Reversed?

One of the most encouraging aspects of early-stage fatty liver disease is its potential for reversal through lifestyle interventions. If you've recently learned about your diagnosis or are concerned about your liver health, it's critical to know that changes you make today can lead to significant improvements tomorrow.

Dietary Changes

Adopting a healthier diet is one of the most effective ways to combat fatty liver disease. The Mediterranean diet, rich in fruits, vegetables, whole grains, healthy fats (like olive oil), and lean proteins (such as fish and chicken), has been shown to reduce liver fat. Conversely, cutting back on sugary foods, refined carbohydrates, and saturated fats can help decrease fat accumulation in the liver. For example, if you follow a low-calorie diet with plenty of vegetables and lean proteins, you can experience a significant reduction in liver fat within just a few weeks.

Regular Exercise

Physical activity is another vital component of liver health. Engaging in regular exercise can help reduce liver fat and improve overall metabolic function. You need to aim for at least 150 minutes of moderate-intensity exercise each week, which can be as simple as brisk walking, cycling, or swimming. If you engage in aerobic and resistance training, you can experience improvements in liver function and a reduction in fat content in the liver (Knudsen, 2022).

Weight Management

If you're overweight or obese, losing even a small percentage of your body weight, 5-10% can have a profound impact on your liver health. This weight loss can significantly reduce liver fat and improve inflammation (Knudsen, 2022).

Monitoring and Support

For those diagnosed with fatty liver, regular monitoring by healthcare professionals can help track progress and make necessary adjustments to treatment plans. Support groups and counseling can also play a significant role in maintaining motivation and ensuring adherence to lifestyle changes.

The road to recovery may not always be smooth, but understanding that early-stage fatty liver can be reversible provides hope. By taking proactive steps towards a healthier lifestyle, you can reclaim your liver health and overall well-being.

Types of Fatty Liver Disease

While both AFLD and NAFLD share a common feature as we

discussed earlier. There are some distinctions between them (Newman, 2018):

Aspect	Alcoholic Fatty Liver Disease (AFLD)	Non-Alcoholic Fatty Liver Disease (NAFLD)
Definition	Fat accumulation in the liver due to excessive alcohol consumption.	Fat accumulation in the liver, not related to alcohol consumption.
Causes	Primarily caused by high alcohol intake.	Associated with obesity, insulin resistance, and metabolic syndrome.
Pathology	The liver's inability to metabolize alcohol leads to fat buildup.	Impaired fat metabolism due to metabolic disturbances.
Stages	Can progress to alcoholic hepatitis and cirrhosis.	Can progress to Non-Alcoholic Steatohepatitis (NASH) and cirrhosis.
Symptoms	Often asymptomatic initially; may include fatigue and abdominal discomfort.	Often asymptomatic; may include fatigue and discomfort in the upper right abdomen.
Risk Factors	High alcohol consumption and a history of alcohol abuse.	Obesity, sedentary lifestyle, unhealthy diet, genetics.
Management	Abstaining from alcohol and nutritional support.	Lifestyle changes (diet, exercise) and weight loss.
Reversibility	Potentially reversible with alcohol cessation.	Early-stage NAFLD is often reversible with lifestyle interventions.

How Genetics, Diet, and Lifestyle Affect Your Liver

Fatty liver disease does not develop in isolation. Various factors interplay to increase the risk of developing AFLD or NAFLD:

1. **Genetics:** Genetics plays a significant role in the susceptibility to fatty liver disease. Certain genetic variants can predispose people to conditions such as obesity, insulin resistance, and lipid metabolism disorders. For example, the *PNPLA3* gene variant is strongly associated with increased liver fat accumulation and progression to NASH. Studies have shown that people carrying this variant are at a greater risk of developing NAFLD, regardless of their alcohol consumption levels (Rich et al., 2018). Understanding your family history can provide insights into your potential risk and help guide preventive measures.
2. **Diet:** Diet is one of the most modifiable risk factors influencing fatty liver disease. Diets high in refined carbohydrates, added sugars, and saturated fats contribute to fat accumulation in the liver. The Western diet, marked by processed foods and sugary beverages, has been linked to a significant increase in NAFLD cases. In contrast, diets rich in whole foods, such as fruits, vegetables, whole grains, and healthy fats (like those found in nuts and fish), can protect against liver fat accumulation (Rich et al., 2018).
3. **Lifestyle Choices:** Physical activity is another critical factor. Sedentary lifestyles are tied to an increased risk of fatty liver disease, as regular exercise helps regulate body weight, improve insulin sensitivity, and enhance fat metabolism. Simple lifestyle changes, like incorporating walking or cycling into your daily routine, can have a significant impact on liver health (Rich et al., 2018).
4. **Comorbidities:** Several comorbidities (when a person has two or more than two diseases at the same time) are closely associated with fatty liver disease, particularly metabolic syndrome. This cluster of

conditions includes obesity, high blood pressure, high blood sugar, and abnormal cholesterol levels. These conditions create a perfect storm for liver health deterioration. For example, people with type 2 diabetes are at a heightened risk for developing NAFLD due to insulin resistance, which directly affects fat metabolism in the liver (Rich et al., 2018).

Understanding Fatty Liver Disease in Children

One of the most concerning trends in recent years is the increasing number of children and teenagers who have fatty liver disease. This condition often relates to obesity, lack of exercise, and poor eating habits, similar to what we see in adults.

Kids with fatty liver disease usually don't show many symptoms, making it hard to spot early. Often, it's only discovered during regular health check-ups or imaging tests. If it's not addressed, pediatric fatty liver conditions can worsen and lead to more serious issues like NASH and liver cirrhosis.

The risk factors for fatty liver in kids are much like those for adults. They include unhealthy food choices, not getting enough exercise, and a family history of liver problems or metabolic conditions. For example, kids who drink a lot of sugary drinks, eat fast food, and snack on processed foods are at a higher risk. Additionally, the increase in screen time and inactivity has made the situation worse, with children spending more time indoors and less time playing outside.

It's crucial to recognize and tackle fatty liver disease in children early on. Making lifestyle changes can lead to big improvements in liver health and overall well-being. Schools and communities can help by promoting healthier habits, encouraging physical activity, and educating families about nutrition. For instance, programs that increase access to healthy foods in schools or that offer after-school activities focused on active play can make a real difference.

Now that we've established a foundation, let's delve into the importance of recognizing the signs and symptoms that can lead to early detection.

2

Recognizing the Signs

In the journey to understanding fatty liver disease, one of the most integral steps is recognizing its signs and symptoms. Many people may not realize they have fatty liver disease until it progresses to a more serious stage, which is why awareness is key. The liver, often referred to as the body's silent workhorse, can develop significant issues without causing noticeable symptoms in its early stages. However, by learning to recognize the symptoms associated with this health illness, you can take proactive measures to address your liver health before it reaches a critical point.

This chapter will delve into the common symptoms of fatty liver disease, emphasizing their significance and encouraging readers to be attentive to their bodies. We will explore both the subtle signs that may easily be overlooked and the more pronounced symptoms that can indicate a progression of the disease.

Symptoms to Watch For

Fatty liver often hides in plain sight during its early stages, as it usually doesn't show symptoms. The liver is a robust organ that can keep functioning even with fat accumulation, so you might not notice anything is wrong until things get worse. And when symptoms finally do show up, they're often pretty vague. This sneaky quality highlights why regular check-ups and liver health screenings are vital, especially for those at risk. Early detection is key to preventing further complications and managing the condition effectively.

Fatigue and Weakness

One of the first and most common signs of fatty liver disease is ongoing fatigue. This feeling of tiredness can linger even after a full night's sleep, making everyday activities feel more strenuous. When the liver struggles to process nutrients and energy efficiently, your overall energy levels may take a hit (Fowler, 2009).

Discomfort or Pain in the Upper Right Abdomen

Another signal to watch for is discomfort or pain in the upper right side of your abdomen, where the liver is situated. This sensation can vary from mild aches to sharp pain and is often mistaken for digestive issues. Since the liver has very few nerve endings, any inflammation or swelling from fatty liver disease can result in discomfort in the surrounding areas (Fowler, 2009). For example, a person can feel a persistent pressure on their side, mistakenly attributing it to digestive troubles when it could be an early indicator of liver problems.

Unexplained Weight Loss

While many people with this disease face weight gain, some might notice unexpected weight loss. This can happen if the body struggles to metabolize fats and carbohydrates properly, leading to an overall reduction in body mass. If weight loss occurs without any changes in diet or exercise, it's important to reach out to a healthcare professional (Fowler, 2009).

Jaundice

Jaundice is a more serious symptom that may develop as fatty liver disease progresses. It is characterized by a yellowing of the skin and eyes, which occurs when the liver can no longer effectively process bilirubin—a waste product produced during the breakdown of red blood cells. When bilirubin levels build up in the bloodstream, it can create a distinctive yellow hue (Fowler, 2009).

Swelling in the Abdomen and Legs

As the liver condition advances, it can give birth to complications such as liver cirrhosis, which may cause swelling in the abdomen (ascites) and legs (edema). This occurs when the liver's impaired function leads to fluid retention in the body. You may notice that their abdomen feels bloated or tight, or they may find their shoes fitting more snugly due to swelling in their feet and ankles. This symptom can be especially concerning, as it often indicates that the liver is struggling significantly (Fowler, 2009).

Changes in Skin Texture

People with fatty liver may also experience changes in skin texture, such as the development of spider angiomas (small, spider-like blood vessels) or palmar erythema (redness of the palms). These skin changes can signal liver dysfunction and may become more pronounced as the disease progresses (Fowler, 2009).

Cognitive Issues

Cognitive impairment, often referred to as "brain fog," can also be a symptom of compromised liver function. People may struggle with concentration, memory, and mental clarity. This cognitive decline can result from the accumulation of toxins in the bloodstream when the liver is not functioning properly (Fowler, 2009). For instance, someone may find themselves frequently forgetting appointments or struggling to focus on tasks they once completed easily. These cognitive challenges can impact everyday life, making it essential to recognize them as potential signs of liver issues.

Increased Blood Sugar Levels

Fatty liver disease can also result in insulin resistance, which, in turn, results in increased blood sugar levels and potentially diabetes. Symptoms, such as frequent urination, increased thirst, and unexplained hunger can arise. This is particularly concerning, as it highlights the interplay between fatty liver disease and metabolic health (Fowler, 2009).

Nausea and Loss of Appetite

You may also experience gastrointestinal symptoms, such as nausea and diminished appetite. This can result from the liver's inability to produce bile, which is required for digesting fats. Over time, this can lead to significant weight loss and nutritional deficiencies (Fowler, 2009).

When to See a Doctor

Recognizing when to seek medical advice about liver health is the most important step, especially if there is a risk of developing a fatty liver. Given the often asymptomatic nature of the early stages of this condition, you may not realize they need to consult a healthcare professional. Understanding the right time to reach out can lead to timely diagnosis and effective management.

Tips for Talking to Healthcare Professionals

1. **Recognizing symptoms:** If you experience any signs commonly linked to fatty liver disease, such as persistent tiredness, discomfort in the abdomen, or noticeable changes in skin tone (like jaundice), seeking advice from a healthcare professional is required. While these signs may stem from a variety of health-related issues, do not disregard them, especially if they are new occurrences or have progressively worsened.
2. **Genetic predisposition to liver conditions:** Should you have a familial background of this disease or related conditions that may impact liver health, such as diabetes or obesity, you must engage your physician in this dialogue. A family history can elevate your risk for fatty liver disease, making proactive monitoring advisable. For example, if a close relative has been diagnosed with non-alcoholic fatty liver disease (NAFLD), consider scheduling regular check-ups to assess your liver function, even if you feel perfectly fine at the moment.

Why Regular Check-Ups Matter

Routine physical examinations are essential for identifying asymptomatic cases of fatty liver disease. In these consultations, healthcare providers can perform various evaluations, including:

- **Physical assessment:** A physician may look for indicators of liver problems, such as jaundice, liver enlargement, or abdominal swelling.
- **Monitoring blood pressure and weight:** Regular assessments of blood pressure and weight can help identify risk factors associated with fatty liver.
- **Evaluation of liver function:** Liver function tests measure the levels of enzymes in the blood (such as ALT and AST), revealing any potential liver inflammation or damage. Elevated enzyme levels may require further investigation.

By establishing a consistent routine with your healthcare professional, you can stay informed about your liver health and address any potential issues without delay.

Understanding Blood Tests and Screening Guidelines

Now is the time to understand the diverse blood tests and screening guidelines crucial to your liver health. Here are some essential points to consider:

1. **Liver Function Tests (LFTs):** Liver function tests encompass a range of blood tests designed to evaluate liver health. These tests gauge enzymes, proteins, and substances generated by the liver, offering insights into its functionality. Elevated levels

of liver enzymes, primarily alanine aminotransferase (ALT) and aspartate aminotransferase (AST), may suggest liver inflammation and often indicate fatty liver disease (Fletcher and Sissons, 2023). Should the results present abnormalities, your healthcare provider might advise further testing, such as imaging studies or even a liver biopsy.

2. **Imaging techniques:** Alongside blood tests, imaging studies can be instrumental in assessing liver health. Ultrasound is a frequently employed method to identify fatty liver, as it can visualize lipid deposits within the liver. Alternative imaging modalities, like CT scans or MRIs, may be used for more comprehensive evaluations, especially if there are concerns about liver damage or other complications.
3. **Guidelines for screening:** The American Association for the Study of liver conditions recommends routine screenings for people with risk factors, such as obesity, type 2 diabetes, or metabolic syndrome (Zhang et al., 2023). Generally, this process involves a combination of blood tests and imaging studies to assess liver health. For instance, should you be diagnosed with metabolic syndrome, your healthcare provider might recommend annual screenings to keep a close eye on any liver-related developments.
4. **Interpreting results:** Comprehending the results of any tests and screenings is also important. If your physician brings up elevated liver enzymes or other concerning findings, don't hesitate to inquire further. Understanding what these results signify about your health will empower you to make educated decisions regarding lifestyle adjustments or additional testing.

The Importance of Early Detection

From the outset, we've underscored the importance of early detection. But why is it so crucial? The sooner a condition is recognized, the broader your options become for reversing liver damage and enhancing overall well-being:

Stopping Disease Progression

Fatty liver disease often evolves through various stages, starting from simple steatosis (fat accumulation) to non-alcoholic steatohepatitis (NASH), which can subsequently lead to severe conditions like liver fibrosis, cirrhosis, or even liver cancer. Early detection enables timely interventions that have the potential to halt or even reverse this progression.

Lifestyle Adjustments

When liver disorder is identified, healthcare professionals can guide patients in making vital lifestyle adjustments. These modifications may include dietary changes, tailored exercise programs, and weight management strategies.

Monitoring Related Conditions

Fatty liver disease can intersect with comorbid conditions such as obesity, diabetes, and elevated cholesterol levels. Early detection presents an opportunity for more effective monitoring and management of these interrelated health challenges. For example, when a patient receives an NAFLD diagnosis, their healthcare provider may assess blood sugar levels and cholesterol, facilitating a holistic approach to their health.

Empowering Through Education

Early detection marks a significant opportunity for patient education. Gaining a clear understanding of your diagnosis allows you to engage actively in managing your health. Resources detailing fatty liver disease can empower you to make informed choices regarding your lifestyle and treatment alternatives.

Cutting Healthcare Expenses

Identifying fatty liver at an early stage can also lead to lower healthcare costs over time. Treating advanced liver disease frequently becomes more complicated and expensive, often involving hospital stays, surgeries, or liver transplants. Conversely, early intervention through lifestyle changes can significantly reduce these expenses.

1. **Influence of lifestyle choices:** Certain personal decisions can heighten your susceptibility to liver diseases, including excessive alcohol intake, lack of physical activity, and poor dietary habits. If you find yourself in these situations, initiating a discussion with your healthcare provider about maintaining liver health is beneficial.
2. **Variations in weight:** Sudden or unexplained changes in your weight could signal potential liver health issues. If you encounter significant weight fluctuations without any deliberate changes to your eating habits or physical exercise, it's important to consult with your doctor.
3. **Importance of regular health assessments:** Consistent health screenings play a vital role in the early discovery of fatty liver disease. During routine assessments, physicians often evaluate general health

and may conduct liver function tests. If you have risk factors like obesity, diabetes, or high cholesterol (hyperlipidemia), regular examinations can reveal any emerging concerns promptly. For instance, an annual physical examination can provide valuable information about liver enzymes and overall liver well-being, allowing for timely interventions when needed.

With a clearer understanding of the signs, we'll explore the diagnostic journey that can provide you with the answers you need.

Exercise: Reflect on Your Liver Health

Take a few moments to reflect on your health and well-being. Write down three signs or symptoms mentioned in the chapter that you or a loved one has experienced. After noting these symptoms, consider the following questions to deepen your understanding and awareness of fatty liver disease:

Reflection on Symptoms

- What was your initial reaction when you or a loved one experienced these symptoms?
- Did you attribute these symptoms to any specific causes, or did you dismiss them as something minor?

Understanding the Implications

- How do you think these symptoms could relate to overall liver health?
- Have you discussed these symptoms with a healthcare professional? If not, what has held you back from doing so?

Instructions:

- Take your time to reflect on each question.
- Write down your thoughts and responses in a journal or a separate sheet of paper.
- Consider sharing your reflections with a trusted friend or family member to facilitate a supportive conversation about health awareness.

3

The Science of Fatty Liver

Fatty liver disease may seem worrisome, but understanding how it develops helps make the science behind it clearer and more manageable.

In this chapter, we'll break down the biological processes that lead to liver disease and how certain factors, like diet and lifestyle, contribute to the build-up of fat in the liver. With this understanding, you'll be better prepared to grasp the steps needed to reverse or manage the condition.

How Fatty Liver Develops

At its core, fatty liver disease is exactly what it sounds like—the accumulation of excess fat in liver cells. While some fat in the liver is normal, this disease occurs when more than five to ten percent of your liver's weight is fat. But how does this fat get there, and why does it cause problems?

The Role of Fat in the Body

First, let's start with the basics. Fat is a vital part of your body's metabolism. It's a source of energy, and when your body doesn't immediately need the calories you consume, it stores them as fat. Normally, fat is stored in places like your abdomen, hips, and thighs. But under certain conditions, fat can begin to accumulate in organs like the liver.

This build-up typically happens when there is an imbalance in how your body processes fats and sugars. For example, if you eat more calories than your body can burn off, especially from fatty or sugary foods, the extra calories get stored as fat. This can result in fat being deposited in the liver, especially when combined with other risk factors like poor diet, lack of exercise, obesity, or insulin resistance.

Insulin Resistance and Liver Health

One of the primary mechanisms leading to fatty liver conditions is insulin resistance (Health direct, 2019). Insulin is a hormone that helps your body process glucose (sugar) from the food you eat. When you develop insulin resistance, your cells don't respond as well to insulin, making it harder for your body to use glucose for energy. As a result, your body produces more insulin to try and compensate, and this excess insulin signals your liver to start storing more fat.

A classic example is Type 2 diabetes. Many people with insulin resistance eventually develop this condition, and those with Type 2 diabetes are at a much higher risk for developing non-alcoholic fatty liver disease (NAFLD). Essentially, the more insulin-resistant you become, the more fat accumulates in your liver.

What Happens When Your Metabolism Goes Awry

Another contributing factor to the development of fatty liver disease of this health condition is lipid overload. Normally, your liver plays a central role in managing fats (lipids) in your body. It processes fats from the food you eat, converting them into forms that can be used for energy or stored for later use. However, when too much fat enters the liver, whether from your diet or from fat being released from fat stores, the liver struggles to keep up. It starts to store the excess fat within its own cells (Arvind et al., 2000).

Think of your liver like a sponge—it can only absorb so much before it gets saturated. Once it reaches this point, it can no longer function optimally, and the excess fat leads to inflammation and damage to liver cells. Over time, this can progress to more serious conditions, such as steatohepatitis (inflammation of the liver due to fat build-up) and eventually cirrhosis (scarring of the liver).

How Genetics Contribute to Fatty Liver

While lifestyle factors, like diet and exercise, are major contributors to fatty liver disease, genetics can also play a significant role. Some people may be genetically predisposed to accumulating fat in their liver, even if they maintain a relatively healthy lifestyle.

The Impact of Diet on Liver Fat

Your diet plays a direct role in the development of fatty liver disorder. Diets high in refined carbohydrates, sugary beverages, and processed foods are notorious for contributing to fat accumulation in the liver. When you consume more carbohydrates than your body needs, it converts the excess into fat, which is stored not only in fat cells but also in the liver.

For example, consider someone who regularly consumes sugary drinks, like sodas or energy drinks. These beverages contain large amounts of fructose, a type of sugar that is processed primarily by the liver. When consumed in excess, fructose can overwhelm the liver's ability to process it, leading to increased fat production and accumulation in the liver.

On the flip side, a diet rich in fruits, vegetables, lean proteins, and whole grains is less likely to contribute to fat build-up in the liver. Mediterranean-style diets, in particular, have been shown to reduce fat in the liver and improve overall liver health.

Alcohol vs NAFLD: What's The Difference?

While non-alcoholic fatty liver disease (NAFLD) is caused by metabolic factors, alcohol can also play a role in fat accumulation in the liver. When you consume alcohol, your liver processes it, breaking it down into chemicals that can be toxic to your cells. Over time, heavy alcohol consumption can result in alcoholic fatty liver disease (AFLD), which is a separate but related condition.

With AFLD, the liver prioritizes processing alcohol over fat, causing fat to accumulate in liver cells. This is why people with a history of heavy drinking are prone to these diseases, like AFLD, alcoholic hepatitis, and cirrhosis. In contrast, NAFLD develops without the influence of alcohol but shares similar features, such as fat build-up and inflammation.

Diet and Habits for a Healthier Liver

When it comes to managing and potentially reversing compromised liver functioning, diet and nutrition play a pivotal role. Your liver is directly impacted by what you eat, making dietary choices impactful in promoting liver health.

Let's discuss how specific foods and dietary habits can influence fatty liver disease and how you can make adjustments to support your liver's well-being.

Understanding the Connection Between Diet and Fatty Liver Disease

Diet is one of the most important contributors to the development of liver diseases. Poor dietary choices, particularly those high in sugars, unhealthy fats, and refined carbohydrates, can cause excess fat accumulation in the liver. Conversely, a nutrient-rich diet can help mitigate this risk.

The liver's primary role is to process nutrients from the food we eat, but when it is overwhelmed by unhealthy options, it struggles to function optimally. Foods high in saturated fats and added sugars can lead to insulin resistance, a key factor in the progression of liver disorder. Essentially, what you eat can either fuel your liver's health or contribute to its decline.

Foods to Embrace for a Healthy Liver

Making mindful dietary choices is also needed to support liver health (Watson, 2024). Here are some food categories to focus on:

- **Fruits and vegetables:** These are rich in vitamins, minerals, and antioxidants that support liver function.

Aim for a variety of colors on your plate, as different fruits and vegetables provide different nutrients.

- **Whole grains:** Foods like brown rice, quinoa, and whole-grain bread are better options than refined grains. They contain more fiber, which helps regulate blood sugar levels and can prevent fat accumulation in the liver.
- **Healthy fats:** Incorporate sources of healthy fats, such as avocados, nuts, seeds, and olive oil. These fats are anti-inflammatory and can help reduce fat accumulation in the liver. Omega-3 fatty acids, found in fatty fish like salmon and mackerel, are particularly beneficial for liver health, as they help lower liver fat levels and inflammation.
- **Lean Proteins:** Opt for lean protein sources, like chicken, turkey, fish, legumes, and tofu. These provide essential amino acids without the unhealthy fats found in fatty cuts of meat.
- **Legumes and Beans:** Foods, such as lentils, chickpeas, and black beans are rich in fiber and protein, which can help you feel fuller longer and stabilize blood sugar levels. They also support digestive health and help reduce liver fat. We will talk about this in detail in the next chapter.

Foods to Avoid

Just as important as knowing what to eat is understanding what to limit or avoid. Here are some dietary culprits that can contribute to fatty liver disease (Watson, 2024):

1. High sugar intake, especially from fructose found in sugary drinks, can lead to fat accumulation in the liver. Soda, sweetened coffee drinks, and even fruit

juices can be problematic. Instead, you need to opt for water, herbal teas, or drinks without added sugars.

2. White bread, pastries, and many processed foods are often stripped of their nutrients and fiber, leading to rapid spikes in blood sugar. These foods can contribute to insulin resistance and, ultimately, accumulation of fat in the liver. So, choose whole grains whenever possible.
3. These unhealthy fats, found in fried foods, baked goods, and processed snacks, can increase liver fat and inflammation. Always check food labels for partially hydrogenated oils, which indicate trans fats. Stick to healthier fats like those found in olive oil or nuts.

Portion Control and Mindful Eating

Beyond food choices, portion sizes and how you eat can significantly impact liver health. Overeating, even healthy foods, can lead to excess calorie intake, promoting fat accumulation in the liver.

Meal Planning for Liver Health

Creating a meal plan can help you stay on track with your dietary goals. Aim for balanced meals that include a variety of food groups. Here's a simple framework to get you started:

- **Breakfast:** Start your day with a bowl of oatmeal topped with fresh fruits and nuts. This meal is high in fiber and can keep you full longer.
- **Lunch:** Prepare a salad with mixed greens, grilled chicken or chickpeas, a variety of colorful vegetables, and a drizzle of olive oil and lemon juice.

- **Dinner:** Opt for baked salmon with quinoa and steamed broccoli. This meal is rich in omega-3 fatty acids and antioxidants.
- **Snacks:** Choose healthy snacks like carrot sticks with hummus, a small handful of nuts, or Greek yogurt with berries.

Don't forget the importance of staying hydrated. Water is crucial for overall health and helps the liver flush out toxins. Aim for at least eight glasses of water a day. You can also include herbal teas or infused water with lemon or cucumber for a refreshing twist.

The Impact of Lifestyle on Liver Health

When it comes to liver health, our daily habits and lifestyle choices play a significant role. From what we eat and drink to how we manage stress and engage in physical activity, every aspect of our lifestyle can either support or hinder liver function.

Let's explore how various lifestyle factors impact liver health and discover practical strategies for making positive changes.

Physical Activity: Moving for a Healthier Liver

Exercise is a cornerstone of good health, and it's particularly beneficial for your liver. Regular physical activity helps maintain a healthy weight, reduces liver fat, and improves insulin sensitivity—key factors in preventing and managing this condition.

Types of exercise: You don't need to become a gym rat to reap the benefits of exercise. The best approach is to find activities you enjoy and can sustain over time. Here are some options:

- **Aerobic exercise:** Activities, like walking, running, cycling, and swimming can help burn calories and improve cardiovascular health. Aim for at least 150 minutes of moderate-intensity aerobic exercise each week.
- **Strength training:** Incorporating strength training exercises into your routine helps build muscle mass and boosts metabolism. You don't need fancy equipment; bodyweight exercises, like squats, push-ups, and lunges are effective.
- **Flexibility and balance:** Activities in the form of yoga and tai chi not only improve flexibility but also reduce stress, which can have a positive impact on liver health. Plus, these practices can help you stay active as you age.

Maintaining a Healthy Weight

Being overweight or obese is one of the primary risk factors for developing fatty liver disease. Excess body fat, particularly around the abdomen, is linked to increased liver fat and inflammation.

Weight management strategies: Achieving and maintaining a healthy weight doesn't have to be complicated. Here are some tips:

- **Set realistic goals:** You can aim for gradual weight loss (one to two pounds per week) rather than drastic changes. Small and sustainable changes are more likely to stick.
- **Keep a food diary:** Tracking what you eat can help you identify patterns and make adjustments. Apps like *MyFitnessPal* or *simple pen-and-*paper methods can work wonders.

- **Practice mindful eating:** Listen to your body's hunger cues and savor each bite. Eating slowly can help you feel more satisfied and prevent overeating.

Managing Stress

Chronic stress can have a surprising impact on liver health. Stress triggers the release of hormones like cortisol, which can lead to unhealthy eating habits, increased alcohol consumption, and even a lack of exercise.

You need to find effective ways to manage stress for overall well-being and liver health. Here are some strategies:

- **Mindfulness and meditation:** Practicing mindfulness or meditation for just a few minutes each day can help reduce stress levels. Focus on your breath or try guided meditations available through apps like Headspace or Calm.
- **Physical activity:** As mentioned earlier, exercise is a powerful stress reliever. Whether it's a brisk walk or a yoga class, moving your body can help clear your mind.
- **Connect with others:** Don't underestimate the power of social connections. Talking to friends or family members about your feelings can provide support and help alleviate stress.

Sleep Quality Matters

Quality sleep is often overlooked when discussing liver health, but it's critical. Poor sleep patterns can disrupt metabolic processes, leading to weight gain and insulin resistance, both of which contribute to illness.

Improving sleep hygiene: Here are some tips to improve your sleep quality:

- **Create a sleep routine:** Go to bed and wake up at the same time each day to regulate your body's internal clock.
- **Limit screen time:** Try to avoid screens (phones, computers, TV) for at least an hour before bedtime. The blue light emitted can interfere with your ability to fall asleep.
- **Create a relaxing environment:** Make your bedroom conducive to sleep by keeping it dark, cool, and quiet. Consider using blackout curtains, earplugs, or a white noise machine.

Always consult with a healthcare professional before taking new supplements or medications, particularly if you have pre-existing liver conditions. Natural doesn't always mean safe, and some herbal supplements can be harmful to the liver.

Finally, regular check-ups with your healthcare provider are vital for monitoring liver health. Routine blood tests and assessments can catch potential problems early, allowing for prompt interventions.

With a solid grasp of the science, we can now explore how nutrition serves as medicine in managing and reversing fatty liver disease.

Activity Time: Liver Lab - Your Personal Experiment

Instructions:

1. Using the knowledge you've gained about the nutritional aspects of liver health, design a meal plan for the day. Make sure to include breakfast, lunch,

dinner, and snacks that are beneficial for liver function.

2. Choose one week to implement your meal plan. Keep track of how you feel physically and emotionally throughout the week.
3. If you're reading this with friends or family, discuss your meal plan and findings with them. Consider doing a taste test with different liver-friendly recipes!

Meal Plan Template

Breakfast:

- **Dish Name:**
- **Ingredients:** (e.g., oatmeal, berries, nuts)
- **Nutritional Benefits:** (e.g., high in fiber, antioxidants)

Lunch:

- **Dish Name:**
- **Ingredients:** (e.g., grilled chicken salad with leafy greens, tomatoes, and olive oil)
- **Nutritional Benefits:** (e.g., lean protein, healthy fats)

Dinner:

- **Dish Name:**
- **Ingredients:** (e.g., baked salmon with quinoa and steamed broccoli)
- **Nutritional Benefits:** (e.g., omega-3 fatty acids, fiber)

Snacks:

- **Snack 1:** (e.g., carrot sticks with hummus)
    - **Nutritional Benefits:** (e.g., low-calorie, high in vitamins)
- **Snack 2:** (e.g., a piece of fruit)
    - **Nutritional Benefits:** (e.g., natural sugars, hydration)

After the week, take a moment to reflect on the following questions:

1. How did you feel physically and mentally during the week? (Consider energy levels, mood, and any digestive changes.)
2. What was the easiest part of sticking to your meal plan?
3. What challenges did you face, and how did you overcome them?
4. Did you discover any new favorite recipes or ingredients that you want to continue using?

4

The Diagnostic Journey

Realizing that something might be wrong with your liver can feel overwhelming, but understanding what comes next can help ease those concerns. The journey to diagnosing fatty liver disease consists of a combination of medical tests, evaluations, and conversations with medical professionals. Many people don't realize they have fatty liver disease until they go in for a routine check-up or notice subtle changes in their health.

Nowadays, modern diagnostic tools can offer a clear picture of what's happening with your liver.

In this chapter, we'll walk you through the tests and procedures used to diagnose fatty liver disease so you know what to expect and how to best prepare for it.

How Fatty Liver is Diagnosed

Detecting fatty liver disease doesn't follow a one-size-fits-all approach. There are various methods doctors use to confirm the presence of fat in the liver, evaluate any potential damage, and determine the stage of the disease. Here's a breakdown of the most common diagnostic tools and procedures:

Blood Tests (Liver Function Tests)

One of the first steps in diagnosing fatty liver disease is often a routine blood test. Your doctor may order a liver function test (LFT), which measures the levels of specific enzymes and proteins in your blood produced by your liver. While blood tests can't directly diagnose fatty liver, they can reveal signs of liver inflammation or damage.

For example, elevated levels of alanine aminotransferase (ALT) or aspartate aminotransferase (AST) can suggest liver inflammation (Juo & Livingston, 2019). However, it's important to note that normal enzyme levels don't always mean your liver is perfectly healthy, and elevated levels don't necessarily confirm fatty liver disease. Your doctor will use these results alongside other tests to get a fuller picture.

Imaging Tests

Once blood tests indicate possible liver issues, imaging tests are usually the next step. These non-invasive procedures allow doctors to get a detailed view of your liver to detect the presence of fat.

- **Ultrasound:** The most commonly used imaging test for diagnosing fatty liver disease is an abdominal ultrasound. This test is painless and involves a technician gliding a small device over your abdomen to create images of your liver using sound waves. Ultrasound can show whether fat is present in the liver, but it can't distinguish between simple fatty liver and more advanced forms like NASH (Non-Alcoholic Steatohepatitis).

- **FibroScan:** Similar to an ultrasound, a FibroScan measures liver stiffness by using sound waves. This test is useful because it can assess both the amount of fat and the degree of liver stiffness (fibrosis), which indicates scarring. FibroScan is often used to monitor people with known liver conditions, but it can also be used in initial diagnosis (Juo & Livingston, 2019).
- **CT scan and MRI:** For a more detailed view, doctors may use computed tomography (CT) scans or magnetic resonance imaging (MRI). Both can detect fat deposits in the liver and provide a clearer image than an ultrasound (Juo & Livingston, 2019). However, these tests are typically more expensive and not always necessary unless the doctor suspects more severe liver damage or complications.

Liver Biopsy

A liver biopsy is considered the most definitive way to diagnose fatty liver and assess its severity. However, it's also the most invasive diagnostic procedure. During a liver biopsy, a small sample of your liver tissue is removed and examined under a microscope. This test can confirm the presence of fat, inflammation, and scarring (fibrosis) in the liver.

Liver biopsies are typically reserved for cases where the diagnosis isn't clear from blood tests or imaging, or when the doctor needs to determine the severity of liver damage, particularly in suspected cases of NASH. For example, someone who has persistently high liver enzyme levels and unclear imaging results may be advised to undergo a biopsy to assess the degree of liver scarring.

While the idea of a biopsy might sound intimidating, the procedure is often quick and done under local anesthesia. Recovery time is usually short, though there may be some mild discomfort afterward.

Transient Elastography

Transient elastography is a non-invasive test that measures the stiffness of your liver using sound waves. It's similar to FibroScan but offers more detailed information about the degree of fibrosis (scarring) in the liver. Stiffer liver tissue suggests a higher degree of fibrosis, indicating the disease may have progressed to a more advanced stage. This test is useful for monitoring disease progression over time, especially in patients already diagnosed with NAFLD or NASH.

For example, if you've been diagnosed with fatty liver disease and are making lifestyle changes to improve your liver health, transient elastography can help your doctor track the effectiveness of those changes and catch any progression early on.

Blood Markers for Fibrosis

In some cases, doctors may use specific blood tests designed to assess liver fibrosis without the need for a biopsy. These tests measure certain proteins and substances that indicate scarring in the liver, such as the Fibrosis-4 (FIB-4) index or the NAFLD fibrosis score. While these tests are not perfect, they can help doctors decide whether a patient is at higher risk for advanced liver illness and whether more invasive tests like a biopsy are necessary (Cox et al., 2021).

For example, if a patient's blood tests show high fibrosis scores, the doctor may order additional imaging tests or a biopsy to confirm the extent of liver damage.

Genetic Testing and Risk Assessments

Genetic testing is becoming another tool in the diagnostic process. Certain genetic variations can make you more susceptible to fatty liver issues, even in the absence of traditional risk factors, like obesity or diabetes. For instance, people with variations in the PNPLA3 gene may have a higher risk of developing NAFLD. Genetic testing can help identify those at higher risk, particularly in families where liver disease is common (Newman, 2018).

Making Sense of Your Results

Once you've gone through the diagnostic process for fatty liver disease, the next step is understanding what those test results actually mean. Medical jargon and complex numbers can be difficult, but breaking them down into simple terms can help make sense of your liver health status. From liver enzyme levels to imaging scans, knowing how to interpret these results gives you a clearer picture of where you stand and what actions might be necessary moving forward.

Let's explore the main components of your results and what they could indicate about your liver.

Blood Tests: What Do Those Numbers Mean?

One of the first tests you may encounter is the liver function test (LFT), which measures levels of liver enzymes and proteins in your blood. While the term "liver function" can make it sound like this test tells you how well your liver is working overall, it actually focuses on detecting liver damage or inflammation. Here's a breakdown of the most common indicators:

- **ALT (Alanine Aminotransferase):** This enzyme is usually present in liver cells, and elevated levels can suggest liver cell damage. Normal ALT levels range from seven to fifty-six units per liter of blood (Cleveland Clinic, 2021). If your ALT level is higher than normal, it can indicate fat buildup in the liver or inflammation. For example, if you have an ALT reading of 65, your doctor may explain that this suggests mild liver inflammation, possibly due to fatty liver. However, they'll likely combine this information with other tests before drawing conclusions.
- **AST (Aspartate Aminotransferase):** Similar to ALT, AST is another enzyme that signals liver damage when elevated. The normal range for AST is about five to forty units per liter (Davis & Memon, 2024). Elevated AST may also indicate issues beyond the liver, like muscle damage, which is why it's often evaluated alongside ALT.
- **Bilirubin:** This substance is produced during the breakdown of red blood cells and is processed by the liver. High levels of bilirubin can indicate liver dysfunction or blockages in the bile ducts, though fatty liver alone doesn't typically cause elevated bilirubin.

Understanding these numbers is important, but it's also important to remember that mildly elevated liver enzymes don't always mean serious liver disease. Sometimes, factors, like exercise or even certain medications can raise these levels temporarily.

Imaging Tests: Seeing Inside Your Liver

If your liver function tests show abnormalities, your doctor may suggest an imaging test like an ultrasound, CT scan, or

MRI. These scans provide a picture of your liver and help determine whether there's any fat accumulation, scarring, or other changes.

- **Ultrasound findings:** The ultrasound report may mention terms like "hepatic steatosis" or "bright liver" both of which suggest the presence of excess fat in the liver. While this can confirm fatty liver disease, it doesn't provide details on the severity. A person diagnosed with "moderate steatosis" based on their ultrasound means that they have a noticeable fat buildup, but additional tests are needed to assess the extent of liver damage.
- **FibroScan results:** If you undergo a FibroScan, your report will include a score that reflects your liver's stiffness (measured in kilopascals, or kPa). A high score (greater than 7 kPa) indicates that there's likely fibrosis, or scarring, in your liver (Foucher, 2006). Severe fibrosis may suggest that the condition has progressed to NASH (Non-Alcoholic Steatohepatitis), a more serious form that can lead to cirrhosis over time.
- **CT scan or MRI:** These more advanced imaging methods give clearer and more detailed images of your liver than an ultrasound. Your doctor may refer to "fatty infiltration" in your liver on the report, which confirms the presence of fat.

Liver Biopsy: What to Expect

- **Steatosis:** This term refers to fat accumulation in the liver. Biopsy results may specify whether the amount of fat is mild, moderate, or severe. Even in cases of severe steatosis, lifestyle changes can help reduce fat levels over time, especially in the early stages.

- **Inflammation:** Your biopsy report may also mention inflammation, which suggests irritation and injury to liver cells. In the context of fatty liver, inflammation can mean the disease has progressed to NASH, a more severe condition (Fletcher, 2022).
- **Fibrosis and Cirrhosis:** Biopsy results that mention fibrosis indicate the presence of scarring in the liver. Early-stage fibrosis can often be reversed with lifestyle changes, but more advanced scarring, known as cirrhosis, is permanent and requires more intensive management. For example, if your biopsy results show stage 2 fibrosis, this indicates moderate scarring but may still be reversible if addressed promptly (Fletcher, 2022).

Understanding Risk Scores: Fibrosis and NAFLD Scores

For those at risk of advanced liver disease, doctors may calculate specific risk scores using blood tests and other data. Two of the most common are the FIB-4 and NAFLD fibrosis scores.

- **FIB-4 Score:** This score combines information from your blood tests (such as liver enzymes) with your age to estimate your risk of liver fibrosis. A low FIB-4 score suggests minimal or no fibrosis, while a higher score indicates that further testing, such as a biopsy or FibroScan, might be necessary. For instance, if your FIB-4 score comes back as 1.5, your doctor may reassure you that this suggests a low risk of advanced fibrosis. On the other hand, a score of 3.0 or higher might prompt your doctor to investigate further for potential scarring (Imai et al., 2023).

- **NAFLD Fibrosis score:** Similar to FIB-4, the NAFLD fibrosis score is another tool that uses blood test results, body mass index (BMI), and age to evaluate your risk of fibrosis. A low score typically suggests minimal risk, while a high score indicates a need for further evaluation (Imai et al., 2023).

Both of these scores help doctors decide whether you need more invasive testing or simply regular monitoring to keep your liver health on track.

Remember that no single test gives a full picture of your liver's health. Doctors typically combine the results from various tests —blood tests, imaging, biopsies, and risk scores to get a comprehensive understanding of your condition.

For example, if your liver enzymes are mildly elevated, your ultrasound shows moderate fat accumulation, and your FIB-4 score is low, your doctor may diagnose you with early-stage NAFLD. Afterward, they will recommend lifestyle changes. On the other hand, if your biopsy shows severe fibrosis, your doctor may discuss more intensive treatment options to prevent further liver damage.

Preparing for Medical Appointments

Once you've gone through diagnostic tests and received your results, the next critical step is having an open and effective conversation with your healthcare provider. Navigating medical consultations can sometimes feel daunting, especially when dealing with a condition which may require long-term lifestyle adjustments or additional tests.

However, with the right approach, you can make the most out of these consultations and feel more confident in managing your liver health.

Preparation: Questions Matter

Before heading into your consultation, take some time to prepare. Having a list of questions ready can help ensure that you cover all the important points during your appointment. This is especially crucial if you feel concerned or worried by medical jargon or if the results of your liver tests are unclear. Writing down your concerns or questions in advance can also make the conversation smoother.

Here are some key questions you might consider asking:

- What stage is my fatty liver disease, and what does it mean for my health?
- What lifestyle changes do you recommend to improve my liver health?
- Are there specific foods or exercises I should avoid?
- What are the risks if I don't address the condition now?
- How often should I come in for follow-up appointments or tests?

Being proactive with these kinds of questions will help you get the answers you need. For example, if your doctor tells you that you're in the early stages of non-alcoholic fatty liver disease (NAFLD), you can ask how much improvement you can expect with dietary changes.

Understand Your Options: Treatment and Lifestyle Recommendations

During the consultation, your doctor will likely present a plan for managing your condition. For most people with fatty liver, lifestyle changes are the first and most crucial line of defense. Expect your doctor to emphasize weight loss if necessary, as even a five to ten percent reduction in body weight can have a significant impact on liver health. Exercise, diet modifications, and perhaps alcohol reduction (in cases of alcoholic fatty liver disease) will likely be discussed.

An example of a lifestyle recommendation might be to follow a Mediterranean-style diet rich in fruits, vegetables, whole grains, and healthy fats like olive oil.

Building a Relationship with Your Doctor

One of the most important aspects of navigating medical consultations is building a good rapport with your doctor. Liver malfunctioning can require long-term management, so it's essential that you feel comfortable asking questions and expressing concerns.

Let's say your doctor recommends regular follow-ups every six months to monitor your liver function. You may feel anxious about ongoing testing or unsure about the progression of your disease. It's okay to voice those concerns. A good doctor will take the time to explain the reasoning behind their recommendations, helping you feel more at ease.

It's also worth noting that liver disease doesn't always progress predictably. Some patients see considerable improvement with lifestyle changes, while others may experience complications despite best efforts. Staying engaged in conversations with your healthcare provider ensures that you're well-informed of your current health status and any changes that may arise over time.

Becoming Your Own Best Advocate

While doctors provide essential medical expertise, you are ultimately the most important advocate for your health. If something doesn't make sense, ask for clarification. If you feel that your concerns are being dismissed or your doctor isn't taking the time to address your questions, it will be worth considering a second opinion.

For example, if your doctor suggests that your liver disease isn't serious enough to warrant lifestyle changes, but you've read about the potential risks of letting it progress, don't hesitate to push for more information. Ask about what you can do proactively to prevent complications, like cirrhosis or liver cancer down the road.

In addition, if you have other health conditions that can complicate your liver disease (such as diabetes or high blood pressure), make sure your doctor is aware of them. These conditions are often interlinked and managing one can benefit the others. A collaborative approach between you and your healthcare team will give you the best chance at managing your liver health effectively.

Making the Most of Follow-Up Appointments

Follow-up consultations are just as important as your initial diagnosis appointment. Fatty liver condition is a dynamic one that can improve or worsen depending on various factors, including adherence to lifestyle changes, weight management, and even genetics. Regular follow-ups give your doctor the opportunity to reassess your condition and adjust treatment recommendations accordingly.

In between visits, it's a good idea to track your progress. For instance, if you've made dietary changes or started exercising regularly, take note of how you're feeling. *Are you losing weight? Do you have more energy? Is your digestion improving?* These observations can provide valuable information during your follow-up visits. Your doctor may ask whether you've noticed any improvement in symptoms or overall well-being, and having concrete answers can help them tailor the next steps in your treatment plan.

In some cases, follow-up appointments may involve additional blood tests or imaging to monitor your liver's response to interventions. If your results show improvement, your doctor may encourage you to continue with your current routine. On the other hand, if your condition hasn't improved or has worsened, they may suggest more aggressive interventions, such as medications or even referral to a liver specialist.

Utilizing Other Healthcare Resources

Beyond your regular visits to the doctor, you may also be referred to other healthcare professionals to support your journey toward better liver health. For instance, a registered dietitian can help you create a personalized meal plan that promotes liver health. An exercise physiologist, on the contrary, can design a workout routine suited to your physical abilities and condition.

Let's say you're struggling to make dietary changes, and your doctor refers you to a dietitian. The dietitian will help you understand how to reduce unhealthy fats and sugars in your diet while still enjoying flavorful meals. They will provide practical suggestions, such as substituting white bread for whole grain or using olive oil instead of butter. This kind of tailored support can make the lifestyle adjustments seem less daunting and more achievable.

Additionally, if your liver illness has progressed, you may work with a hepatologist—a specialist in liver diseases. A hepatologist can provide more in-depth care, especially in complex or advanced cases.

Armed with your diagnosis, it's time to dive into the science of fatty liver disease and understand its underlying mechanisms in the next chapter.

Activity: Map Your Health Journey

- **Gather your supplies:** Grab a piece of paper, a pen, and any coloring tools (markers, colored pencils, etc.) if you want to add visual elements. This can be as simple or creative as you'd like!
- **Draw the timeline framework:** Draw a horizontal line across the page. This line represents the journey of your liver health over time. Mark the far-left end of the line as your *starting point*, representing your health journey up to this moment. The far-right end represents *future health goals*, where you want to be in managing your liver health.
- **Identify your starting point:** Reflect on where you are right now in your liver health journey. Think about: Write a brief note about this at the beginning of your timeline, noting any relevant dates, recent discoveries, or feelings you have about your starting point.
- **Plot significant milestones:** As you move from left to right, mark key milestones you have encountered or expect to reach. For each milestone, add a brief description and, if you like, a date or approximate timeline. This will give you a clear view of the steps you've taken and those still ahead.

- **Define your future goals:** On the right side of the timeline, mark your liver health goals. These can be: Be specific with each goal. For example: "Lower ALT/AST levels by next check-up" or "Incorporate a liver-friendly meal plan by the end of the month." The more concrete these goals are, the easier it will be to track and celebrate your progress.

5

Nutrition as Medicine

When it comes to liver health, the old saying "you are what you eat" couldn't be more accurate. Nutrition plays a crucial role in maintaining optimal liver function and can even help reverse some of the damages caused by conditions like fatty liver disease.

In this chapter, we'll learn how food acts as medicine for the liver and highlight specific "superfoods" that can help keep your liver in tip-top shape.

Superfoods for Liver Health

So, what exactly are superfoods? They're nutrient-rich foods that are particularly beneficial for health and well-being. While no single food can cure fatty liver disease or guarantee perfect health, certain superfoods can support liver function and aid in detoxification, making them valuable allies on your journey to better liver health.

Leafy Greens: The Power of Chlorophyll

Let's start with leafy greens. You can think of spinach, kale, and Swiss chard. These vibrant veggies are packed with chlorophyll, which helps detoxify the liver by neutralizing heavy metals, chemicals, and pesticides. Incorporating leafy greens into your diet can enhance your liver's ability to cleanse itself (Watson, 2024).

How to enjoy them: Try adding a handful of spinach to your morning smoothie, tossing some kale into a stir-fry, or creating a delicious salad with mixed greens, tomatoes, and avocado. The options are endless, and you'll benefit from their nutrients while enjoying a variety of flavors.

Cruciferous Vegetables: The Detox Heroes

Cruciferous vegetables, like broccoli, Brussels sprouts, and cauliflower, are also excellent for liver health. They contain compounds that help increase the liver's detoxification enzymes, which play a key role in eliminating toxins from the body.

A simple recipe: Consider making roasted Brussels sprouts tossed with olive oil, garlic, and a sprinkle of sea salt. Not only are they tasty, but they also provide a satisfying crunch while promoting liver detoxification.

Berries: Antioxidant Powerhouses

Berries—blueberries, raspberries, and cranberries are delicious and are loaded with antioxidants, particularly anthocyanins, which have been shown to protect the liver from damage and reduce inflammation. These compounds support liver health by improving liver fat levels and enhancing the liver's overall function (Watson, 2024).

Snack ideas: Snack on a handful of berries, blend them into a smoothie, or add them to your oatmeal for a nutrient boost. They're versatile and can easily fit into your daily routine.

Nuts: Healthy Fats for Liver Support

Nuts, particularly walnuts and almonds, are a great source of healthy fats, vitamin E, and omega-3 fatty acids. Walnuts, for example, contain high levels of the amino acid arginine, which helps detoxify ammonia, a waste product that can accumulate in the body and cause damage to the liver (Watson, 2024).

Incorporate nuts: A handful of nuts makes for a perfect snack or can be sprinkled on salads and yogurt for added crunch and flavor. Just remember to watch your portion sizes, as nuts are calorie-dense.

Fatty Fish: Omega-3 Rich Delights

Fatty fish, like salmon, sardines, and mackerel, are rich in omega-3 fatty acids, which can help reduce liver fat and inflammation. Omega-3s have been shown to improve liver health by promoting healthy fat levels in the liver (Watson, 2024).

Cooking tip: Aim to include fatty fish in your diet at least twice a week. You can grill salmon, add canned sardines to salads, or bake mackerel for a delicious and nutritious meal.

Garlic: The Flavorful Detoxifier

Garlic is not only a fantastic flavor enhancer but also a powerful superfood for liver health. It contains sulfur compounds that activate liver enzymes that are responsible for flushing out toxins. Additionally, garlic can help reduce liver fat and improve overall liver function (Watson, 2024).

Use garlic creatively: Add minced garlic to stir-fries, pasta sauces, or roasted vegetables to enjoy its benefits while enhancing the taste of your meals.

Avocado: Creamy Goodness

Avocado is another superfood that supports liver health. It's high in healthy monounsaturated fats and contains compounds like glutathione, which help the liver detoxify harmful substances. Research has suggested that avocados may even help reduce liver damage and improve liver function (Cherney, 2023).

How to enjoy avocado: Spread avocado on whole-grain toast, mix it into salads, or create a creamy avocado dressing for your meals. Its versatility makes it easy to incorporate into your diet.

Olive Oil: A Heart-Healthy Fat

Olive oil is a staple of the Mediterranean diet and is considered a healthy fat. It's rich in antioxidants and can help lower liver enzyme levels while promoting overall liver health. Studies have shown that replacing saturated fats with healthy fats, like those found in olive oil, can benefit liver function (Cherney, 2023).

Cooking with olive oil: Use olive oil as a base for salad dressings, drizzle it over roasted vegetables, or use it for cooking at low to medium heat. Just be mindful not to heat it to its smoke point, as that can create harmful compounds.

Turmeric: The Golden Spice

Turmeric contains curcumin, a compound with powerful anti-inflammatory and antioxidant properties. This spice has been shown to protect the liver from damage and may help improve liver function by promoting the regeneration of liver cells (Kunnumakkara et al., 2023).

Incorporate Turmeric: You can add turmeric to curries, smoothies, or even golden milk. Its vibrant color and warm flavor can liven up various dishes.

Green Tea: The Liver's Ally

Green tea is packed with antioxidants, particularly catechins, which have been linked to improved liver function and fat reduction in the liver. Drinking green tea regularly may help support liver health and prevent fatty liver disease.

A simple habit: Consider swapping your afternoon coffee for a cup of green tea. Not only will you enjoy its soothing qualities, but you'll also benefit from its liver-protective properties.

How to Build a Liver-Friendly Diet

Creating a dietary plan tailored for liver health can feel restrictive and over-tiring, but it doesn't have to be. With a bit of guidance and an understanding of what works best for your liver, you can easily implement changes that promote overall well-being. The goal here is to craft a balanced and sustainable eating plan that nourishes your body while supporting liver function.

Embrace Whole Foods

At the foundation of any healthy dietary plan should be an emphasis on whole, unprocessed foods. These foods provide essential nutrients and antioxidants that the liver needs to function optimally. Think fresh fruits and vegetables, whole grains, lean proteins, and healthy fats.

Incorporating high-quality protein sources is essential for liver health. Protein helps repair liver tissues and produces enzymes that facilitate metabolic processes. Opt for lean proteins like fish, poultry, beans, lentils, and tofu.

Meal idea: A quinoa bowl with black beans, diced tomatoes, corn, and avocado delivers plant-based protein and packs in fiber, which aids digestion and supports liver health.

Limit Saturated Fats and Refined Carbs

While healthy fats are beneficial, it's important to limit saturated fats and refined carbohydrates, which can contribute to fat accumulation in the liver. Foods high in saturated fats include fatty cuts of meat, full-fat dairy products, and processed snacks. Refined carbs like white bread, pastries, and sugary cereals can lead to insulin resistance and worsening liver health.

Tip: Swap out refined carbs for whole grains. Instead of white rice, choose brown rice or quinoa. Rather than reaching for white bread, go for whole-grain options. This simple switch can have a significant impact on your liver health.

Stay Hydrated

Hydration is often overlooked but is crucial for liver health. Water helps the liver flush out toxins and aids in digestion.

Aim to drink at least eight to ten cups of water a day, and remember that hydration doesn't just come from beverages—fruits and vegetables with high water content can also contribute to your daily intake.

Fun Idea: Try infusing your water with slices of lemon, cucumber, or mint for a refreshing twist. This will make drinking water more enjoyable and provide additional nutrients.

Limit Alcohol Consumption

If you have fatty liver, it's best to limit or eliminate alcohol entirely. Alcohol can exacerbate liver inflammation and damage, making it more difficult for the liver to recover. If you choose to drink, moderation is essential. While the selection of non-alcoholic alternatives has significantly improved in recent years, it's still important to enjoy them in moderation due to the sugars and additives often used to replicate the flavor.

Example: If you enjoy social gatherings where drinks are present, consider opting for non-alcoholic alternatives, like sparkling water with a splash of fruit juice or herbal teas.

Mind Your Portion Sizes

Portion control is very important in any dietary plan. Eating large portions, even healthy foods, can lead to excess calorie intake and contribute to weight gain, which is a risk factor for fatty liver disease.

Tip: Use smaller plates to help control portion sizes. This simple trick can make a meal feel more satisfying without overloading your plate.

Plan Balanced Meals

Aim for a balance of macronutrients at each meal. This means including a good mix of proteins, healthy fats, and carbohydrates. A well-rounded meal not only fuels your body but also helps maintain stable blood sugar levels, reducing the risk of insulin resistance.

Sample meal: For dinner, consider baked salmon with a side of roasted sweet potatoes and steamed broccoli. This meal provides protein, healthy fats, and fiber-rich carbohydrates—all supportive of liver health.

Consider Meal Timing

Some research suggests that meal timing can play a role in liver health (McCommis & Butler, 2020). Eating regular and balanced meals throughout the day can help regulate blood sugar levels and reduce liver fat. Avoid skipping meals, as this can lead to overeating later.

Practice: Try to establish a routine where you eat three balanced meals and two healthy snacks each day. This can help stabilize your energy levels and keep your metabolism active.

Finally, if you're unsure where to start or need personalized recommendations, consider working with a registered dietitian or nutritionist. They can provide tailored advice based on your specific health needs, dietary preferences, and lifestyle.

Navigating Diets: Myths vs. Facts

When it comes to dietary advice, the world can feel like a confusing maze of information, especially regarding liver health and fatty liver disorder. With so many diets claiming miraculous results, you need to separate fact from fiction.

Here, we'll debunk common myths about diets related to liver health and provide facts to help you make informed decisions for your well-being.

Myth 1: All Fats Are Bad for Your Liver

Fact: Not all fats are created equal! While it's true that saturated and trans fats can harm your liver, healthy fats, like those found in avocados, nuts, seeds, and olive oil are actually beneficial. These fats provide essential fatty acids and can help reduce inflammation.

Myth 2: You Need to Go on a Strict Diet to Heal Your Liver

Fact: While making dietary changes is crucial for liver health, it doesn't mean you have to follow a strict or overly restrictive diet. Instead of labeling foods as "good" or "bad," focus on moderation and balance. A sustainable approach will yield better long-term results.

Rather than cutting out entire food groups, try incorporating more whole foods into your meals. If you enjoy a piece of cake occasionally, savor it without guilt. The key is to balance indulgences with healthier choices throughout the week.

Myth 3: You Can Detox Your Liver with Juice Cleanses

Fact: Your liver is already equipped to detoxify your body. The idea that you need to do a juice cleanse or a detox diet to "cleanse" your liver is misleading. These diets can often be low in essential nutrients and may even do more harm than good.

Instead of a juice cleanse, opt for a diet rich in fruits and vegetables, whole grains, and lean proteins. This way, you provide your liver with the nutrients it needs to function effectively without putting it through the stress of extreme dieting.

Myth 4: Carbs Are Bad for Your Liver

Fact: Carbohydrates are an essential part of a balanced diet, but the type of carbohydrates you consume matters. Refined carbs, like those found in white bread, sugary snacks, and pastries—can contribute to liver fat accumulation. Instead, focus on complex carbohydrates, such as whole grains, fruits, and vegetables.

When you choose carbs, think "whole" over "refined." A bowl of oatmeal topped with fresh berries is a delicious way to start your day while supporting liver health.

Myth 5: All Alcohol is Dangerous for Liver Health

Fact: While excessive alcohol consumption is detrimental to liver health, moderate alcohol intake may not be harmful for everyone. The key is moderation. For some people, especially those with fatty liver disease, it may be best to avoid alcohol altogether.

Myth 6: You Can Spot-Reduce Fat in Your Liver with Certain Foods

Fact: Unfortunately, there's no magic food that can target fat loss in your liver. The body loses fat uniformly rather than in specific areas. The best approach is to focus on an overall healthy lifestyle, including a balanced diet and regular exercise.

Myth 7: Only Obese Individuals Develop Fatty Liver Disease

Fact: While obesity is a main risk factor for fatty liver disorders, it's not the only one. People of all body types can develop fatty liver, especially if they have other risk factors like diabetes, high cholesterol, or a sedentary lifestyle.

Myth 8: Supplements Can Cure Fatty Liver Disease

Fact: While some supplements may support liver health, no miracle pill can cure fatty liver disease. Relying solely on supplements without addressing diet and lifestyle changes is ineffective.

If you're considering supplements, consult your healthcare provider first. They can recommend appropriate supplements that can complement your diet and help with liver health, like milk thistle or omega-3 fatty acids. But, remember that they should be part of a comprehensive approach to health, and nutrition from food is always best.

Nutrition is just one piece of the puzzle; let's now examine how regular exercise can further enhance your liver's well-being in the upcoming chapter.

Myth vs. Fact Quiz

Before moving on to the next chapter, below are several statements regarding fatty liver disease. For each statement, determine whether it is a myth or a fact.

1. **Statement 1:** "Fatty liver disease only affects people who are overweight."
   - Myth/Fact

2. **Statement 2:** "Alcohol consumption is the only cause of fatty liver disease."
    - Myth/Fact
3. **Statement 3:** "Fatty liver disease can lead to serious health complications, including liver cirrhosis."
    - Myth/Fact
4. **Statement 4:** "People with fatty liver disease often have no symptoms until the condition is advanced."
    - Myth/Fact
5. **Statement 5:** "Diet and exercise can reverse fatty liver disease."
    - Myth/Fact
6. **Statement 6:** "All fatty liver diseases are the same; there's no difference between alcoholic and non-alcoholic fatty liver disease."
    - Myth/Fact

6

The Power of Exercise

When we think about improving our health, diet often takes center stage, while exercise may seem like an afterthought. However, exercise plays a direct role in supporting liver health, especially for those dealing with or at risk for fatty liver disease.

This chapter explores the undeniable link between physical activity and a healthy liver, demonstrating how movement can be a powerful tool in your wellness arsenal.

How Exercise Helps Your Liver Heal

Engaging in regular physical activity offers a myriad of benefits, and liver health is no exception. For those with fatty liver disease, exercise acts as a catalyst for positive change, helping to reduce liver fat, improve liver function, and enhance overall metabolic health. Let's break down how exercise can make a real difference.

Reducing Liver Fat

One of the most significant benefits of exercise is its ability to reduce liver fat. Research indicates that even moderate physical activity can lead to substantial reductions in liver fat, especially in people with Non-Alcoholic Fatty Liver Disease (Fowler, 2009). Engaging in aerobic exercises, like brisk walking, swimming, or cycling can effectively help burn excess fat stored in the liver.

Enhancing Insulin Sensitivity

Exercise also plays a crucial role in improving insulin sensitivity, which is vital for metabolic health. Insulin resistance is a common issue among those with fatty liver disease, contributing to the accumulation of fat in the liver. Regular physical activity helps your body use insulin more effectively, which can lead to better blood sugar control and a reduction in liver fat (Fowler, 2009).

Boosting Overall Metabolism

Regular exercise can rev up your metabolism, making it easier to maintain a healthy weight or lose excess pounds. Weight loss can help reduce liver fat and improve liver health.

Stress Reduction and Emotional Well-being

Exercise isn't just beneficial for the body; it's also a powerful tool for mental health. Physical activity releases endorphins, the body's natural mood lifters, which can help alleviate stress and anxiety. For those coping with the challenges of managing a chronic condition like fatty liver disease, this emotional boost can be invaluable.

Finding an exercise routine you enjoy, whether it's dancing, hiking, or joining a local sports team—can make it easier to stick with it. When exercise feels more like fun and less like a chore, you're more likely to maintain it in the long run.

Creating a Holistic Approach

Integrating exercise into your lifestyle is about creating a holistic approach to liver health. Combine physical activity with a balanced diet, proper hydration, and adequate sleep to support your liver's needs. This comprehensive approach can amplify the benefits of each component, leading to better overall health.

Creating Your Ideal Exercise Routine

When it comes to improving liver health through exercise, having a well-structured workout plan can make all the difference. An effective workout plan helps you stay motivated and ensures that you're getting the right mix of aerobic activity, strength training, and flexibility work.

Let's look at how to create a workout plan that fits your lifestyle and supports your liver health:

Set Clear and Achievable Goals

The first step in creating an effective workout plan is to set clear and achievable goals. Whether you want to lose weight, improve your endurance, or simply feel more energetic, having specific goals will guide your planning and keep you motivated.

For example, instead of vague goals, like "I want to exercise more," consider setting specific targets, such as "I will walk 30 minutes a day, five days a week."

Aerobic Exercise

Aerobic exercise can lower liver fat and improve cardiovascular health. Aim for at least 150 minutes of moderate-intensity aerobic activity each week. Here are some ideas to include in your plan:

- **Walking:** A simple yet effective way to get moving. You can start with short walks and gradually increase the duration and pace.
- **Cycling:** Whether it's on a stationary bike or outdoors, cycling can be a fun way to boost your heart rate.
- **Swimming:** A low-impact option that's easy on the joints, making it ideal for those with mobility issues.
- **Dancing:** Join a dance class or simply dance at home—whatever gets you moving and having fun!

Tip: Break your weekly aerobic activity into manageable chunks. For example, you can aim for thirty minutes of walking five times a week or fifty minutes three times a week.

Strength Training

Strength training can help you build muscle, boost metabolism, and improve overall body composition. You can go for two to three sessions per week, focusing on major muscle groups. Here are some effective strength training exercises:

- **Bodyweight exercises:** Push-ups, squats, lunges, and planks can be done anywhere and require no equipment.
- **Resistance bands:** These are portable and provide a great way to add resistance without heavy weights.

- **Weights:** If you have access to dumbbells or weight machines, consider incorporating them into your routine.

A simple strength training plan can involve two sets of 10-15 repetitions for each exercise, focusing on different muscle groups on different days (e.g., upper body one day, lower body the next).

Flexibility and Balance

Flexibility and balance are often overlooked but are crucial for overall fitness, especially as we age. Incorporate activities that promote flexibility and balance into your weekly routine:

- **Yoga:** A fantastic way to improve flexibility, decrease stress, and enhance overall well-being. Look for beginner classes in your community or follow online sessions.
- **Stretching:** Dedicate a few minutes after each workout to stretch major muscle groups.
- **Balance exercises:** Simple exercises, like standing on one leg or walking heel-to-toe can help improve balance.

Listen to Your Body

As you embark on your exercise journey, always listen to your body. Start slowly, especially if you're new to exercise or have been inactive for a while. Pay attention to any signs of discomfort and adjust your plan as needed.

For instance, if you experience pain while doing a particular exercise, don't hesitate to modify it or choose an alternative that feels better for you.

Consistency is key to seeing results, so stick to your workout plan as closely as possible.

Track Your Progress

Keeping track of your workouts and progress can provide motivation and help you stay accountable. Consider using a journal, a fitness app, or a simple calendar to record your workouts, track your achievements, and celebrate milestones along the way. If you notice that you can now walk a mile faster than when you started, take a moment to acknowledge that progress!

Consult with Professionals

If you're unsure where to start or have specific health concerns, consulting with a fitness professional or a health-care provider can help you. They can help tailor a workout plan to your unique needs and ensure you're exercising safely.

Tips to Stay Active and Motivated

Staying motivated on your fitness journey, especially when it comes to improving liver health, can sometimes feel like a challenge. However, keeping your spirits high and tracking your progress can make a significant difference.

Find Your 'Why'

Understanding why you want to improve your liver health through exercise is very helpful for maintaining motivation. Whether it's to boost your energy levels, reduce liver fat, or simply feel better overall, having a personal reason can help you push through those days when motivation wanes.

If your goal is to have more energy to play with your kids or grandkids, keep that in mind when you feel like skipping a workout. Visualizing your 'why' can help reignite your motivation.

Setting clear and achievable goals can create a sense of direction and purpose. Break down larger goals into smaller and manageable milestones to make the journey feel less daunting and more rewarding.

Create a Workout Schedule

Having a structured workout schedule can help you stay accountable. Designate specific days and times for your workouts and treat them like important appointments you cannot miss. Consistency will make exercise a part of your routine, and it'll be easier to stick with it.

Tip: You can use a calendar or a planner to block out your workout times and mark them as completed when you finish. This visual representation of your commitment can be very motivating.

Again, track your progress as it will help you keep aware and motivated.

Celebrate Small Wins

Don't forget to celebrate your milestones! Acknowledging your progress, whether big or small, can reinforce positive behavior and keep you motivated.

Consider treating yourself to something special after reaching a goal, like new workout gear or a massage. Celebrating achievements helps you associate exercise with positive experiences.

Mix It Up

To avoid boredom and keep things exciting, mix up your workout routine. Trying new activities or classes can challenge your body in different ways and keep your enthusiasm alive. So, keep things fresh and engaging, and don't be afraid to mix up your activities. Try new classes, explore different parks for walking, or switch up your strength training routine every few weeks.

Find a Workout Buddy

Exercising with a friend or family member can boost motivation and accountability. Having a workout buddy makes the experience more enjoyable, and you're less likely to skip a workout when someone else is counting on you.

Stay Flexible

Life can be unpredictable, and sometimes, your plans may not go as scheduled. It's essential to stay flexible and not be too hard on yourself if you miss a workout or have to modify your routine.

If you can't fit in a longer workout, you can replace it with a short 10-minute session. Or you can incorporate physical activity into your daily tasks, like taking the stairs instead of the elevator. Remember, every bit counts!

As we enhance our physical health, it's vital to consider the emotional aspect of our journey. Let's discuss the intersection of mental health and liver disease.

Activity: Move Your Liver - Create Your Own Fitness Plan!

Instructions:

- Take a few minutes to reflect on your current physical activity level. How much time do you spend exercising each week? What types of exercise do you enjoy? Write your thoughts in a journal.
- Think about what you want to achieve regarding your liver health. Use the SMART criteria (Specific, Measurable, Achievable, Relevant, Time-bound) to create a goal. For example: "I will walk for 30 minutes, five days a week, for the next month to improve my liver health."

Design Your Weekly Exercise Plan: Weekly Exercise Plan Template

- Based on the information provided in the chapter, create a balanced exercise routine that includes aerobic exercise, strength training, and flexibility/balance activities. Use the template below to outline your plan:
- If you have friends or family members interested in improving their health, share your exercise plan with them. Consider forming a small group to work out together, discuss your goals, and encourage each other.

Track Your Progress: Tracking Template

- Use a journal, app, or calendar to track your workouts. Note how you feel after each session, any changes in your energy levels, and progress towards your goals.

Reflect on Your Experience

- At the end of the week, take a moment to reflect on your exercise routine. What worked well? What would you like to change for the next week? Write down your reflections.
- Did you achieve your exercise goals?
- How did your mood and energy levels change throughout the week?
- What was the most enjoyable part of your routine?
- Are there any new activities you want to try next week?

7

Mental Health and Liver Disease

As we delve into the connection between mental health and liver disease, we need to recognize how our emotional well-being influences our physical health, particularly the liver. The liver is not just a silent workhorse in our bodies; it's also affected by our stress levels, emotional health, and overall mental state.

In this chapter, you will see how stress impacts liver health, the mechanisms behind this relationship, and practical strategies to manage stress for a healthier liver.

How Stress Affects Your Liver

Stress is an inevitable part of life, but how we manage it can make a big difference to our overall health. When we experience stress, our body goes into a heightened state of alertness, producing hormones, like cortisol and adrenaline (WebMD Editorial Contributors, 2022). While this response can be helpful in short bursts, like during a deadline at work or a tough workout, chronic stress can wreak havoc on our bodies, including our liver.

The Physiological Connection

Chronic stress can give birth to various physiological changes that may contribute to liver problems. Elevated levels of cortisol, often called the "stress hormone," can promote fat accumulation in the liver, leading to conditions like fatty liver disease. Additionally, stress can result in increased blood sugar levels and insulin resistance, further exacerbating liver-related issues (Vere et al., 2009).

Breaking The Stress-Health Cycle

Stress can create a vicious cycle: unhealthy coping mechanisms like poor diet and lack of exercise can lead to weight gain and liver issues, which, in turn, can increase stress levels. It's a cycle that can be difficult to break, but understanding it is the first step toward better liver health.

Emotional Well-Being and Liver Function

Research has shown that emotional well-being can significantly impact liver function (Vere et al., 2009). Conditions, such as anxiety and depression can affect the way our body metabolizes nutrients and eliminates toxins, further stressing the liver. This connection underscores the importance of addressing mental health as part of a holistic approach to liver care.

Practical Stress-Management Techniques

Fortunately, there are effective strategies for managing stress that can help protect liver health. Here are some simple, practical techniques to consider:

- **Regular exercise:** Physical activity is a natural stress reliever. It not only boosts endorphins (our body's feel-good hormones) but also improves overall health, including liver function. Whether it's a brisk walk, a dance class, or yoga, find an activity you enjoy and make it a regular part of your routine.
- **Balanced diet:** Nourishing your body with a balanced diet rich in fruits, vegetables, whole grains, and lean proteins can provide the nutrients your liver needs to function optimally.
- **Social connections:** Spending time with friends and family can alleviate stress and promote emotional well-being. Building a support network allows for sharing experiences and seeking comfort during challenging times.
- **Professional help:** If stress becomes overwhelming, seeking help from a mental health professional can be invaluable. Therapy can offer coping strategies and a safe space to explore emotions.

Mindfulness and Meditation

Mindfulness and meditation are impactful tools for managing stress and enhancing overall well-being, especially for people dealing with liver health issues. By incorporating these practices into your daily routine, you can cultivate a greater sense of calm, improve emotional resilience, and support your liver health. Here are some practical techniques to get you started:

Breathing Exercises

One of the simplest forms of mindfulness practice is focusing on your breath. This technique can be done anywhere, anytime, and it's a great way to ground yourself in the present moment. Here's how to do it:

- **Find a comfortable position:** Sit or lie in a quiet place. You can close your eyes or soften your gaze.
- **Inhale deeply:** Breathe in slowly through your nose, allowing your abdomen to rise as you fill your lungs with air. Count to four as you inhale.
- **Pause:** Hold your breath for a count of four.
- **Exhale slowly:** Release your breath through your mouth, counting to six as you let it all out. Imagine stress and tension leaving your body with your breath.
- **Repeat:** Continue this cycle for a few minutes, focusing solely on your breath and letting any distracting thoughts drift away.

Guided Meditation

Guided meditation encompasses listening to a narration that leads you through a meditation session, often incorporating visualizations and affirmations. You can find many free guided meditations online or through apps. Here's a basic framework to try:

- **Choose a comfortable space:** Sit or lie down in a comfortable position where you won't be disturbed.
- **Select a meditation:** Look for a guided meditation focusing on relaxation or stress relief. You can choose one specifically tailored for liver health if available.
- **Set the scene:** Close your eyes and take a few deep breaths to settle in. Allow yourself to focus solely on the voice guiding you.
- **Engage your senses:** As you listen, try to visualize the imagery presented and engage your senses. For instance, if the guide mentions a peaceful beach,

imagine the sound of the waves, the warmth of the sun, and the scent of salt in the air.
- **Conclude gently:** When the meditation ends, take a moment before opening your eyes to notice how you feel. Slowly transition back to your day.

Mindful Eating

Mindful eating is a fantastic way to connect with your body and improve your relationship with food—important for maintaining liver health. Here's how to practice it:

- **Eliminate distractions:** Sit down for your meal away from screens and noise. This helps you focus on the food in front of you.
- **Observe your food:** Before you begin eating, take a moment to observe your food. Notice the colors, textures, and aromas. This engages your senses and prepares you for a mindful experience.
- **Take smaller bites:** Chew your food slowly and savor each bite. Pay attention to the flavors and how the food feels in your mouth.
- **Listen to your body:** Notice when you start to feel full and stop eating when you reach that point. This practice fosters a healthier relationship with food and can prevent overeating.

For example, if you're having a salad for lunch, take time to appreciate the fresh ingredients. As you eat, focus on the crunch of the lettuce and the tanginess of the dressing. This will help you enjoy your meal more fully and reduce stress around eating.

Daily Mindfulness Practice

Incorporating mindfulness into your daily life doesn't have to be limited to formal meditation. Here are a few simple ways to be more mindful throughout your day:

- **Mindful walking:** As you walk, pay attention to each step. Feel your feet connect with the ground, notice the rhythm of your breath, and observe your surroundings without judgment.
- **Mindful moments:** Set reminders throughout your day to pause and take a few deep breaths, or simply take a moment to appreciate your surroundings—whether it's the beauty of nature, a friendly smile, or the aroma of your favorite beverage.
- **Gratitude practice:** At the end of each day, reflect on three things you are grateful for. This practice can shift your mindset toward positivity and reduce stress.

While commuting, instead of scrolling through your phone, you can take a few moments to observe the scenery around you. This simple act can bring a sense of peace and connection to your environment.

Building a Support System

When it comes to managing liver health, having a strong support system can make a world of difference. Dealing with a health condition can sometimes feel isolating, but connecting with others who understand your journey can provide comfort, encouragement, and valuable insights. Let us learn how to build a solid support network and the types of support that can help you thrive.

Connect with Healthcare Professionals

Your first line of support should be your healthcare team. Establishing a good rapport with your doctors, nutritionists, and mental health professionals is very important. They are there to offer you medical guidance and help you navigate the complexities of liver disease. During your connections:

- **Open communication:** Be honest about your symptoms, concerns, and lifestyle. The more your healthcare team knows, the better they can support you. Don't hesitate to ask questions or seek clarification about your treatment plan.
- **Follow-up visits:** Regular check-ups can help track your progress and make necessary adjustments to your care. They also offer a chance to discuss any new symptoms or challenges you're facing. If you're feeling overwhelmed with your dietary restrictions, talk to your nutritionist. They will provide practical meal ideas or coping strategies. This, in turn, will make the process feel less daunting and easier to handle.

Lean on Family and Friends

Family and friends can be an invaluable source of emotional support. They can help you stay motivated, provide companionship, and assist with day-to-day challenges. Here's how to involve them in your journey:

- **Educate them:** Share information about fatty liver disease with your loved ones. The more they understand what you're going through, the better they can support you. Consider having an open conversation about how your condition affects your daily life and what support you need from them.

- **Invite participation:** Encourage your family and friends to join you in healthy activities, such as cooking nutritious meals together or going for walks. This helps you stay on track and fosters a sense of togetherness.

For example, if you're trying to adopt a healthier diet, ask a friend to join you for a cooking night where you prepare liver-friendly recipes. This creates a fun atmosphere and makes it easier to stick to your goals.

Seek Out Support Groups

Joining a support group can be incredibly beneficial, as it connects you with others who share similar experiences. Support groups provide a platform to share stories, advice, and coping strategies.

- **In-person or online:** Look for local support groups in your area, or consider joining online forums and communities. Many organizations focused on liver health offer resources for connecting with others.
- **Participate actively:** Attend meetings regularly and engage in discussions. Sharing your experiences can be cathartic, and you may find that others resonate with your journey. Listening to their stories can also provide new perspectives and coping techniques.

If you find an online group that meets weekly to discuss liver health topics, don't hesitate to join in. Hearing how others manage their conditions can inspire you and remind you that you're not alone in this journey.

Consider Professional Counseling

If you're feeling particularly worried or anxious about your liver health, consider speaking with a mental health professional. They can help you process your emotions and develop coping strategies.

- **Coping mechanisms:** A therapist can teach you effective techniques for managing stress and anxiety, equipping you with tools to handle the emotional aspects of living with a chronic condition.
- **Safe space:** Therapy offers a confidential environment where you can express your feelings without judgment. This can be particularly beneficial when navigating the ups and downs of your health journey.

If you experience anxiety about your condition or its impact on your life, talking to a therapist can help you work through those feelings and develop a more positive mindset.

With our mental health strategies in place, we can now explore how to manage co-existing conditions that often accompany fatty liver disease.

Activity: Stress Mapping Exercise

- **Objective:** Identify and map out sources of stress to build awareness and confidence in addressing them.
- **Instructions:**
    - Begin with a blank piece of paper and divide it into sections labeled "Work," "Family," "Health," and "Other."
    - Take five to ten minutes to write down specific stressors in each category.

  - Once mapped, circle areas you feel more capable of controlling or addressing.
  - Conclude by choosing one manageable action for each circled stressor.

Gratitude and Reflection Journaling

- **Objective:** Foster emotional well-being and resilience through positive reflections.
- **Instructions**:
  - Write down three things you're grateful for regarding your health or life.
  - Reflect on how gratitude practices impact your emotional state and contribute to liver health.
  - After five to ten minutes, share your reflections in small groups.

8

Managing Co-existing Conditions

Fatty liver disease often doesn't exist in isolation. It's commonly associated with other health conditions, such as diabetes, obesity, high blood pressure, and high cholesterol, which forms a dangerous cycle affecting your overall well-being.

When these conditions overlap, they can compound each other, making it even more challenging to manage each one effectively. However, understanding how these interconnected conditions affect your liver health and learning how to manage them can significantly improve your outcomes.

This chapter will explore how fatty liver condition interacts with common co-existing conditions, starting with diabetes and obesity.

How Fatty Liver Links to Diabetes and Obesity

Fatty liver ailment is strongly tied to both diabetes and obesity. These three conditions often develop together, creating what is known as a "metabolic syndrome," a cluster of conditions that multiplies the risk for heart disease, stroke, and liver damage (Nevola et al., 2023).

Let's dive into how diabetes and obesity are connected to fatty liver disease, and why managing them is crucial for protecting your liver health.

The Link Between Diabetes and Fatty Liver Disease

Diabetes, particularly type 2 diabetes, and fatty liver are closely related. In fact, studies suggest that people with type 2 diabetes are at more risk of developing non-alcoholic fatty liver disease (Huang, 2009). The relationship is a two-way street: fatty liver disease can make it harder to control blood sugar levels, while high blood sugar from diabetes accelerates liver damage.

Here's how it works: in type 2 diabetes, the body becomes resistant to insulin, a hormone responsible for regulating blood sugar. This resistance leads to high levels of glucose in the blood, which can eventually result in excess fat being deposited in the liver. Over time, this accumulation of fat in the liver can cause inflammation and damage, progressing from simple fatty liver (NAFLD) to non-alcoholic steatohepatitis (NASH), and eventually to more severe liver ailments like cirrhosis.

Let's understand it with the help of an example of someone diagnosed with type 2 diabetes. If they're not actively managing their blood sugar levels, they're risking complications, like nerve damage or heart disease, and also increasing their likelihood of liver damage. The liver, overwhelmed by both fat buildup and the effects of high blood sugar, may start to scar or become inflamed, worsening over time.

Obesity and Fatty Liver Disease

Obesity is one of the most common risk factors for fatty liver disease. In fact, up to 90% of people with obesity may have some form of fatty liver (Hashem et al., 2021). Obesity affects liver health by increasing fat deposits in the liver, leading to the same cascade of damage that's seen in diabetes-related fatty liver conditions.

When you carry excess weight, especially around your abdomen, fat sits in fat cells and accumulates in your organs, particularly the liver. This visceral fat contributes to insulin resistance, chronic inflammation, and metabolic dysfunction, all of which further worsen liver problems.

For people who are both obese and diabetic, the risk of liver damage is even higher. Managing both conditions effectively is crucial to halting or reversing the progression of compromised liver issues and functions.

Let us take the case of someone who is both obese and has fatty liver disease. They may struggle with fatigue and abdominal discomfort but not realize that the fat accumulating around their belly is also damaging their liver. If left unchecked, this fat buildup can eventually lead to liver scarring (fibrosis), a precursor to cirrhosis.

The Vicious Cycle of Multiple Conditions

What makes the combination of diabetes, obesity, and fatty liver condition particularly dangerous is that they feed into each other. Obesity leads to insulin resistance, which increases the risk of type 2 diabetes. In turn, both obesity and diabetes cause or worsen fatty liver disease. If the liver is already damaged, managing diabetes becomes more difficult, and the cycle continues.

The metabolic dysfunction underlying these conditions results in higher levels of inflammation, fat accumulation, and oxidative stress in the body, all of which put additional strain on the liver.

The good news is that this cycle can be interrupted through effective lifestyle changes. Diet, exercise, and medical interventions can reduce the impact of both obesity and diabetes on liver health, helping to reverse fatty liver disease at its earlier stages.

Medical Interventions for Managing Multiple Conditions

For those with more advanced fatty liver conditions or severe obesity and diabetes, lifestyle changes alone may not be enough. Medical interventions, such as weight loss surgery (bariatric surgery) or medications that improve insulin sensitivity, may be recommended by a healthcare provider.

- **Weight loss surgery:** In cases of severe obesity, bariatric surgery can dramatically reduce fat deposits in the liver. It has been shown to reverse fatty liver disease in many cases by promoting significant weight loss (Laursen et al., 2019).
- **Medications:** Some medications used to treat type 2 diabetes, such as GLP-1 receptor agonists or SGLT2 inhibitors, have been shown to help reduce liver fat (Nevola et al., 2023). Additionally, new treatments are being developed specifically for fatty liver, though they are still in the research phase.

Strategies for Managing Your Health Holistically

Managing co-existing conditions like fatty liver disease, diabetes, and obesity requires a well-rounded and comprehensive approach. You can't treat one without addressing the others. Fortunately, adopting a holistic strategy can yield improvements across the board, positively affecting liver health, blood sugar control, and weight management.

Let us explore how we can manage our health:

Step 1: A Balanced Diet Tailored to Your Needs

Nutrition is the cornerstone of managing your liver health, obesity, and diabetes. However, know that there's no one-size-fits-all diet. Your eating plan should be tailored to your individual health concerns, lifestyle, and preferences. That being said, there are universal principles that are beneficial for managing these conditions together, as we have already discussed in detail:

- focus on whole foods
- Mediterranean diet
- reduce sugars and refined carbohydrates
- prioritize protein for weight management

Step 2: Regular Physical Activity

Exercise is another main factor in keeping your liver healthy, diabetic-free, and away from obesity. Regular physical activity has a wide range of benefits, from improving cardiovascular health to reducing liver fat and enhancing blood sugar control. Engaging in consistent exercise will help you burn calories and increase insulin sensitivity, allowing your body to manage blood sugar levels more effectively and reduce fat buildup in the liver.

Cardiovascular exercises, such as walking, jogging, swimming, or cycling can significantly improve overall health. Even low-impact activities, like brisk walking, can help reduce liver fat, aid in weight loss, and improve insulin resistance.

Resistance or strength training also plays a major role. Building muscle helps improve metabolism, meaning you'll burn more calories even at rest. Moreover, strength training helps maintain or increase lean muscle mass, which is important for long-term weight management and metabolic health.

Incorporating two to three days of resistance training per week, using free weights, resistance bands, or bodyweight exercises like push-ups and squats can complement cardiovascular exercises. This balance can help in losing fat and support a healthier liver by improving insulin sensitivity.

Step 3: Managing Stress and Mental Health

Mental health is an often-overlooked aspect of managing physical conditions like fatty liver, diabetes, and obesity. Stress can have a direct impact on your health, particularly when it comes to conditions related to metabolism. So, you can incorporate mindfulness exercises.

Step 4: Medical Monitoring and Support

You need to work closely with healthcare professionals to manage these co-existing conditions effectively. Regular check-ups, blood tests, and other forms of monitoring are going to help you catch any worsening symptoms early and adjust your treatment plan as needed.

Your healthcare provider will likely recommend regular blood tests to monitor your liver enzymes, blood sugar levels, cholesterol, and triglycerides.

Step 5: Setting Realistic Goals and Tracking Progress

Managing multiple health conditions requires patience and perseverance. Set small, achievable goals to stay motivated and on track. Whether your goal is to lose a certain amount of weight, reduce your HbA1c (a marker of long-term blood sugar control), or improve your liver enzyme levels, breaking it down into manageable steps will make the process less overwhelming.

Preventing Disease Progression With Lifestyle Changes

Preventing disease progression, especially in the context of co-existing conditions like fatty liver disease, diabetes, and obesity, means you need to adopt a proactive approach. By focusing on regular health screenings, lifestyle modifications, and personalized treatment plans, you can effectively manage their health and stave off complications.

This section will delve into these three critical strategies, highlighting their importance and providing practical insights for implementation.

Regular Health Screenings for Early Detection

Early detection is a game-changer in preventing disease progression. Regular health screenings can help you identify potential complications before they escalate, allowing for timely intervention. This is particularly important for those managing chronic conditions, like liver conditions and diabetes, where early signs of progression may not always be noticeable without medical testing.

Why Regular Screenings Matter

1. Regular screenings can help track liver function through blood tests measuring liver enzymes (like ALT and AST).
2. Regular health screenings can also help detect related health issues, such as hypertension or high cholesterol, which often accompany diabetes and other liver diseases. By addressing these interconnected conditions early, you can reduce the rate of developing cardiovascular disease, a common complication of diabetes and liver issues.
3. Regular visits to healthcare providers allow for a comprehensive assessment of health. This can include screenings for liver ultrasound imaging, blood tests, and monitoring of weight and blood pressure. Building a complete health profile enables tailored treatment plans that address all aspects of an individual's health.

Lifestyle Modifications to Prevent Further Liver Damage

When it comes to preventing disease progression, lifestyle modifications must be taken into account. We have been talking about it time and again only to understand its impact on the liver and overall health.

Personalized Treatment Plans for Complex and Multiple Conditions

Recognizing that each individual is unique is essential for effective disease management. Personalized treatment plans that consider a person's specific health conditions, lifestyle, and preferences can largely improve outcomes and enhance overall well-being.

Collaborative Care Approach

A collaborative approach involving healthcare providers, dietitians, exercise specialists, and mental health professionals ensures that all aspects of a person's health are considered. This holistic method helps in creating a treatment plan tailored to the person's unique needs.

Working with a team of healthcare specialists can offer comprehensive care. For example, a patient with fatty liver and diabetes may benefit from a dietitian's guidance on meal planning, an exercise therapist's support for developing a fitness routine, and a mental health counselor's assistance with stress management.

Regular Reassessment and Adjustment of Treatment Plans

Health is not static; it evolves over time. Therefore, regular reassessment of treatment plans is a must-have. As you make lifestyle changes, your needs and responses to treatment may also change.

Regular follow-ups and health assessments allow healthcare providers to adjust treatment plans based on progress or any emerging health issues. This can include changing medications, adjusting dietary recommendations, or modifying exercise routines.

For instance, a man with obesity and a liver full of fat experiences significant weight loss after implementing lifestyle changes. During a follow-up appointment, his doctor adjusts his medications for diabetes, reducing the dosage due to improved blood sugar levels. This adjustment illustrates the importance of ongoing monitoring and personalization in treatment.

Empowering Individuals through Education

Education has the ability to empower people to take charge of their health. For instance, if you know about your conditions, treatment options, and effective self-management strategies, you can easily foster a sense of agency, confidence, and control.

You can participate in educational workshops or utilize online resources as they can help you better understand your condition. Knowledge about how fatty liver disorder, diabetes, and obesity are interconnected can motivate you to adhere to treatment plans and make informed lifestyle choices.

A community health organization, for example, can offer workshops on managing chronic conditions. By attending it, you can learn about the links between diet and liver health and discover new recipes that align with your dietary needs. Armed with this knowledge, you are going to feel more equipped to manage your health proactively.

Now that we've covered co-morbidities, let's take a closer look at medication and treatment options available for fatty liver disease.

9

Medication and Treatment Options

When we think about taking care of our bodies, we often focus on food choices, exercise, and stress management. But what happens when lifestyle modifications aren't enough? This is where medical interventions and treatments come into play, especially for conditions like fatty liver disease. Understanding the various medication and treatment options available can make a huge difference in managing the disease, making sure that progression is halted or even reversed.

In this chapter, we'll explore current treatments for fatty liver disease, covering medications, therapies, and emerging approaches that healthcare professionals recommend to support liver health.

Current Treatments for Fatty Liver

Currently, there is currently no single "magic pill" to cure fatty liver conditions. However, advancements in medical science are offering promising avenues for managing and treating this condition. The treatment approach largely depends on the type and severity of the disease, as well as the presence of other health issues, like diabetes, obesity, or high cholesterol.

Lifestyle Changes: The First Line of Defense

Before we explore medications, it's important to acknowledge that lifestyle changes are often the first step in treatment. For patients with early-stage NAFLD, doctors typically recommend a combination of weight loss, dietary modifications, and increased physical activity as the primary treatment. This is because reducing liver fat can reverse the early effects of this condition, improving liver function over time.

For example, a patient diagnosed with NAFLD might begin by cutting out processed sugars and unhealthy fats, while also starting a regular exercise routine. With a weight loss of seven percent, they may see a significant reduction in liver fat, leading to improved liver function.

Current Treatments

While lifestyle changes are key, sometimes they are not enough, particularly if you have been diagnosed with more advanced stages of liver condition, like non-alcoholic steatohepatitis (NASH), which can lead to liver fibrosis and cirrhosis. Here's a breakdown of some medications used either directly or indirectly in managing fatty liver:

Vitamin E and Antioxidants

One of the more common treatment approaches for NASH is prescribing Vitamin E. This antioxidant is thought to reduce oxidative stress and inflammation in the liver, both of which are significant contributors to the progression of fatty liver disease.

Why it works: Inflammation is a primary factor in the worsening of fatty liver. By lessening oxidative stress, which is essentially the damage caused by an imbalance of free radicals and antioxidants, Vitamin E can help protect liver cells from further damage (Rees, 2023).

Pioglitazone (Actos)

Pioglitazone, a medication commonly used to treat type 2 diabetes, has shown promise in treating NASH(Lian & Fu, 2021). It works by improving insulin sensitivity, which is often impaired in people with fatty liver disease. When insulin resistance improves, it can reduce liver fat accumulation and inflammation.

Why it works: Insulin resistance is a common problem in people with both diabetes and NAFLD/NASH. By increasing the body's sensitivity to insulin, Pioglitazone helps regulate blood sugar levels, which indirectly lowers fat buildup in the liver (Lian & Fu, 2021).

For example, a patient with both type 2 diabetes and NASH may be prescribed Pioglitazone to manage their diabetes. Over time, their liver health may improve as a side benefit of better blood sugar control.

GLP-1 Receptor Agonists (Liraglutide and Semaglutide)

Originally developed to treat diabetes, GLP-1 receptor agonists, like Liraglutide and Semaglutide are now being explored for their potential in treating liver disorders associated with fat. These medications help lower blood sugar levels and encourage weight loss, which can be beneficial for managing both diabetes and fatty liver disease (Collins & Costello, 2023).

Why it works: Weight loss and keeping blood glucose in check are key strategies for reducing liver fat and inflammation in people with NAFLD. GLP-1 receptor agonists promote weight loss by regulating appetite and slowing gastric emptying, which leads to a reduction in calorie intake (Collins & Costello, 2023).

Obeticholic Acid (OCA)

Obeticholic acid is another promising medication under investigation for treating NASH. It works by activating receptors that reduce liver inflammation and promote fat breakdown. This medication is still undergoing clinical trials but has shown positive results in reducing liver fibrosis and fat accumulation (Shah & Kowdley, 2020).

Why it works: The drug works by activating FXR, a receptor in the liver that regulates bile acid synthesis and transport, fat metabolism, and inflammation (Shah & Kowdley, 2020). By targeting these pathways, obeticholic acid helps reduce the build-up of fat in the liver and slows down the progression of fibrosis (scarring).

In clinical trials, patients treated with OCA showed a significant improvement in liver fibrosis after 18 months of treatment compared to those given a placebo. This makes it a potential treatment option for those with advanced disease (Shah & Kowdley, 2020).

Statins

Though primarily used to lower cholesterol, statins are sometimes prescribed to patients with NAFLD who also have elevated cholesterol levels. Statins help reduce the risk of cardiovascular disease, which is a significant concern for people with fatty liver disease (Egan & Prasad, 2011).

Why it works: People with compromised liver functioning are often at a higher risk for heart disease, so managing cholesterol levels becomes a priority. By reducing cholesterol, statins also help alleviate some of the metabolic complications associated with this disease (Egan & Prasad, 2011).

A patient, for example, with both high cholesterol and NAFLD may be prescribed statins to manage their cardiovascular risk. While statins are not a direct treatment for liver disease, they help manage the broader health issues related to the condition.

Emerging Therapies and What's on the Horizon?

While current treatments for liver disease are primarily focused on managing symptoms and related conditions, ongoing research is paving the way for new therapies. Some promising treatments include:

FXR agonists, such as Tropifexor, are currently being studied for their role in regulating bile acid metabolism and reducing liver inflammation. These drugs may help improve insulin sensitivity and decrease liver fat, making them potential treatments for NASH.

Early studies suggest that FXR agonists can reduce liver fibrosis and inflammation in patients with advanced fatty liver disease. However, these medications are still in the experimental phase, so more research is needed to confirm their efficacy (Yang & Wang, 2023).

FGF19 analogs are another class of drugs being researched for their potential to treat NASH. These medications target metabolic pathways in the liver, reducing fat accumulation and inflammation. In clinical trials, FGF19 analogs have shown promise in reducing liver fat and improving insulin sensitivity in patients with liver condition, although they are still being tested for long-term safety and effectiveness (Yang & Wang, 2023).

The Importance of a Personalized Approach

It's important to recognize that its treatment is not one-size-fits-all. Each person's treatment plan should be tailored based on the severity of their own disease, the presence of co-existing conditions, and how they respond to lifestyle changes and medication. Some patients may respond well to lifestyle modifications alone, while others may require a combination of lifestyle changes and medication.

For instance, a 45-year-old woman with early-stage NAFLD may successfully manage her condition through weight loss and dietary changes. On the other hand, a 60-year-old man with NASH and diabetes may require a more aggressive treatment approach, including medication and ongoing medical monitoring.

Balancing Benefits and Risks of Treatment

When it comes to treating this health disorder, navigating the balance between the benefits and risks of medical interventions is vital. While medications and treatments can offer significant relief and slow disease progression, they also come with potential side effects and considerations.

In this section, we will explore both the positive impacts of current treatments and the potential risks associated with them. Understanding these aspects will help patients and caregivers make informed decisions about their health and treatment options.

The Benefits of Treatment

One of the greatest advantages of medical treatment for fatty liver disease is the ability to slow or even reverse the progression of the condition, particularly in cases of non-alcoholic steatohepatitis (NASH), which can lead to liver fibrosis and cirrhosis. Let's take a closer look at the key benefits of treatment options available today.

Reduction of Liver Fat

A major goal is to decrease the amount of fat accumulated in the liver. This is necessary because excessive fat leads to inflammation and scarring, which can result in liver damage over time. Medications like Pioglitazone and GLP-1 receptor agonists (e.g., Liraglutide and Semaglutide) can be used to reduce liver fat. These treatments are particularly effective for people who also have diabetes or obesity, as they help improve insulin sensitivity and promote weight loss.

Lowering Inflammation

Another key benefit of medical treatments is their ability to reduce liver inflammation, which is a critical factor in the progression of fatty liver. Antioxidants like Vitamin E and medications like Obeticholic Acid (OCA) work by lowering inflammation and oxidative stress within the liver.

Preventing Complications

Untreated fatty liver can lead to more serious liver conditions, including cirrhosis and liver cancer. Medical treatments can help prevent these complications by targeting the underlying causes, such as fat accumulation and inflammation. In addition, medications that address co-existing conditions, like high cholesterol or diabetes, play a role in reducing the overall health risks associated with fatty liver disease.

For example, a patient with NAFLD and high cholesterol may be prescribed statins to manage their cholesterol levels. Not only does this treatment reduce their cardiovascular risk, but it also helps alleviate some of the metabolic complications.

The Risks and Side Effects

While the benefits of treatment are clear, it is equally important to be aware of the potential risks and side effects associated with these medications. Here are some of the common risks to consider:

Side Effects of Medications

As with any medication, treatments for fatty liver disorder can come with side effects, which may vary from mild to severe, depending on the person. For example, Pioglitazone, while effective in reducing liver fat, is associated with weight gain and an increased risk of bone fractures in some people (Lian & Fu, 2021). These side effects may limit its use, particularly for those who are already overweight or at risk of osteoporosis.

Increased Cardiovascular Risks

Some medications used for the treatment, particularly those that address cholesterol levels, can increase the risk of certain cardiovascular events. Statins, for example, while generally considered safe, may cause muscle pain or damage in some individuals (Egan & Prasad, 2011). It's important to balance the benefits of lowering cholesterol with the potential risks, particularly in patients who already have heart disease.

For example, a patient with both fatty liver disease and a history of heart problems may need to be closely monitored while taking statins to ensure that the medication doesn't exacerbate any existing conditions.

Long-Term Unknowns for Emerging Treatments

While newer treatments, like Obeticholic Acid and GLP-1 receptor agonists, have shown promise in clinical trials, the long-term effects of these medications are still being studied. This means that patients using these treatments may face unknown risks as they continue treatment over several years (Shah & Kowdley, 2020).

Weighing the Benefits and Risks: A Personal Approach

One of the key principles in medicine is individualized care, and this is especially important when it comes to treating a serious disease. The benefits and risks of any treatment must be weighed carefully, considering not only the condition of the liver but also the overall health of the individual.

Balancing Risks with Severity of the Disease

In some cases, the risks of a particular medication may be outweighed by the benefits, especially if the patient is in the advanced stages of a liver disorder. For example, a patient with NASH and severe fibrosis can benefit from a more aggressive treatment approach, such as Obeticholic Acid or other experimental therapies, even if they come with some risks. The potential for halting or reversing liver damage may be worth the side effects.

Let us understand it with the help of an example. A patient with stage 3 fibrosis may opt for a trial medication that has shown promising results in halting disease progression, even though the long-term risks of the treatment are not fully understood. This decision would be made in consultation with their healthcare provider, weighing the immediate need to prevent further liver damage against potential side effects.

Considering Co-Existing Conditions

For patients who have other conditions, like diabetes, obesity, or high cholesterol, the treatment plan must also address these co-existing conditions. Medications that improve liver health might also help manage these conditions, but they may also introduce risks that need to be considered.

A patient with NAFLD and diabetes may benefit from a medication like Liraglutide, which not only improves liver health but also aids in weight loss and blood sugar control. However, they would need to monitor their blood sugar levels closely, as this medication could cause hypoglycemia if not properly managed.

The Future of Fatty Liver Disease Treatment

The future of fatty liver disease treatment is one filled with promise as medical research continues to expand our understanding of this increasingly common condition. With the rise of non-alcoholic fatty liver disease (NAFLD) and non-alcoholic steatohepatitis (NASH), the urgency to develop new and more effective treatments is greater than ever. Currently, there are no FDA-approved medications specifically for fatty liver, but exciting advancements in research suggest that this could change in the coming years.

Emerging Medications: Targeting Inflammation and Fibrosis

One of the most promising areas of research is the development of medications aimed at reducing liver inflammation and fibrosis. These two factors play a crucial role in the progression of NAFLD and NASH, leading to more severe complications like cirrhosis and liver failure if left untreated.

Anti-fibrotic Therapies

Currently, several medications targeting liver fibrosis are being tested in clinical trials. One such drug is *Cenicriviroc*, a dual CCR2/CCR5 antagonist that works by blocking specific receptors involved in the inflammatory response in the liver. Early results from trials suggest that Cenicriviroc may slow the progression of liver fibrosis in patients with NASH (Lefebvre et al., 2016).

Anti-inflammatory Medications

Another area of focus is reducing liver inflammation, a key driver of disease progression in both NAFLD and NASH. Drugs, like *Emricasan*, a pan-caspase inhibitor, are being investigated for their ability to reduce liver cell death and inflammation. Though studies are still in the early stages, Emricasan can potentially help halt the inflammatory processes that lead to liver scarring (Yang & Wang, 2023).

Gene Editing and Precision Medicine: A Tailored Approach

As our understanding of genetic factors grows, the concept of gene editing and precision medicine is gaining traction in the treatment of this condition. Precision medicine involves tailoring treatments to a person's genetic makeup, lifestyle, and environment, making it an ideal strategy for liver conditions. This can be influenced by numerous factors.

CRISPR Gene Editing

One of the most exciting possibilities for the future of fatty liver treatment is the potential for gene editing technologies like *CRISPR* (Clustered Regularly Interspaced Short Palindromic Repeats). CRISPR allows scientists to edit specific genes, offering the potential to correct genetic mutations that contribute to fatty liver disease (Xu et al., 2020).

Researchers are currently exploring how CRISPR can be used to modify genes that influence liver fat accumulation and metabolism. Although this technology is still in its infancy, the potential to prevent or even reverse fatty liver disease through gene editing is an exciting prospect.

Precision Medicine in Practice

Precision medicine is already being explored in the context of fatty liver disease. By analyzing a patient's genetic profile, researchers can predict how they may respond to certain treatments or lifestyle interventions. This can also lead to more effective treatment plans that are personalized to each patient's unique biological makeup.

Gut Microbiome and Liver Health: New Frontiers in Treatment

Recent research has also highlighted the critical role of the gut microbiome, the community of bacteria and other microorganisms living in our digestive tract in the development and progression of fatty liver disease. The connection between the gut and liver, often referred to as the *gut-liver axis*, suggests that targeting the microbiome could be a novel way to treat or even prevent fatty liver (Wang et al., 2022).

Probiotics and Prebiotics

Probiotics, which are beneficial bacteria, and prebiotics, which promote the growth of these bacteria, are being studied for their potential to improve liver health by altering the gut microbiome. Early research indicates that probiotics may help reduce liver fat and inflammation by promoting a healthier balance of gut bacteria (Wang et al., 2022).

Fecal Microbiota Transplantation (FMT)

Another intriguing area of research is *fecal microbiota transplantation* (FMT), a procedure in which a healthy person's gut bacteria are transferred to someone with an imbalanced microbiome. FMT has been used successfully to treat conditions like Clostridium difficile infection, and researchers are now exploring its potential for treating liver illnesses, including NAFLD (Wang et al., 2022).

Lifestyle Interventions Enhanced by Technology

While lifestyle changes, such as diet and exercise remain the cornerstone of treating fatty liver, the future will likely see technology playing a greater role in helping individuals maintain these changes over the long term.

Wearable Devices and Health Apps

Wearable devices that track physical activity, heart rate, and sleep patterns are becoming increasingly popular tools for managing chronic diseases, including fatty liver disease. In the future, these devices can be used to monitor liver health in real time, helping you stay on top of your lifestyle goals and receive personalized feedback on your progress.

A patient with NAFLD can use a wearable fitness tracker that syncs with a mobile app designed to monitor liver health. The app can provide real-time data on the patient's physical activity levels, sleep patterns, and diet, offering tailored recommendations to optimize liver health.

Telemedicine and Virtual Coaching

Telemedicine and virtual health coaching are also likely to play a huge role in the future of this disease treatment. These services allow patients to receive ongoing support from healthcare professionals without needing to visit a clinic, making it easier to stick to treatment plans and make necessary lifestyle changes.

The future of fatty liver treatment will likely involve a combination of medications, lifestyle interventions, and emerging technologies. Rather than relying on a one-size-fits-all approach, the focus will shift towards personalized, multifaceted treatment plans that address the unique needs of each patient.

As research continues to advance, we can expect more targeted therapies, improved diagnostic tools, and a greater understanding of how factors like genetics, the gut microbiome, and lifestyle choices contribute to liver health. With these developments, the outlook for people with compromised liver is becoming more hopeful than ever.

With this knowledge, let's talk about how to navigate life while living with fatty liver disease and integrate healthy habits into your daily routine.

10

Living with Fatty Liver Disease

Living with liver disease can feel scary at first, but it's important to remember that with the right lifestyle adjustments, managing the condition is not only possible but can significantly improve your overall health and quality of life. The diagnosis doesn't mean you're helpless; instead, it's a call to action and a chance to reshape your habits and make empowering changes. Whether it's tweaking your diet, incorporating natural remedies, or adopting healthier daily routines, you need to find balance and sustainability.

In this chapter, we'll talk about practical lifestyle adjustments and home remedies that can make a real difference in managing fatty liver disease.

Daily Adjustments for Liver Wellness

One of the most effective ways to manage fatty liver disease is through a balanced and nutrient-rich diet. The liver plays a vital role in processing everything we eat, so what you choose to put on your plate directly impacts your liver health.

Your key focus should be on whole foods, those that are unprocessed or minimally processed. These foods give essential nutrients without the added sugars, unhealthy fats, or artificial ingredients that can strain your liver. Whole grains, fresh fruits, vegetables, lean proteins, and healthy fats from sources like olive oil, nuts, and avocados are excellent options. Avoiding refined carbohydrates, sugary drinks, and high-fat junk foods is essential, as these can contribute to further fat buildup in the liver.

Low Glycemic Index Foods

Choosing foods with a low glycemic index (GI) is particularly helpful for you. The glycemic index measures how quickly a food raises your blood sugar levels. Foods with a high GI, such as white bread, sugary cereals, and processed snacks, cause blood sugar spikes that can worsen insulin resistance, a common issue in those with fatty liver (Coyle, 2023).

Low-GI foods, on the other hand, help maintain stable blood sugar levels, reducing the risk of fat accumulation in the liver. Some excellent low-GI options include whole grains, like quinoa and oats, legumes, most fruits and vegetables, and foods rich in fiber. So, next time, you need to swap out a high-GI breakfast, like a sugary pastry for a bowl of oatmeal topped with fresh berries and a handful of nuts. This simple switch will stabilize your blood sugar and provide fiber, antioxidants, and healthy fats that support liver function.

Supplements and Antioxidants for Liver Health

Your liver is responsible for detoxifying the body, which means it's constantly exposed to oxidative stress. Over time, this stress can damage liver cells and contribute to the progression of liver disorders. Antioxidants (compounds that protect cells from oxidative damage) can help you neutralize these harmful effects and support liver health.

One of the most natural ways to boost your antioxidant intake is through diet. Foods rich in vitamins C and E, along with polyphenols (plant compounds with antioxidant properties), can help lower inflammation and protect the liver.

- **Vitamin C:** Found in citrus fruits, bell peppers, and broccoli, vitamin C is known for its immune-boosting properties and its ability to combat oxidative stress in the liver.
- **Vitamin E:** Nuts, seeds, and leafy greens are excellent sources of vitamin E, which helps reduce liver inflammation and improves liver enzyme levels.
- **Polyphenols:** Green tea is packed with polyphenols that can help you improve liver function and reduce fat deposits in the liver.

Herbal Supplements

Several herbal supplements have been used with the potential to support liver health. While they aren't a cure, some herbs have shown promise in reducing liver inflammation, improving liver enzyme levels, and protecting liver cells.

While the herbs mentioned are known for their liver-supporting benefits, they may not be suitable for everyone. Always consult your healthcare provider before starting any herbal regimen, especially if you are pregnant, breastfeeding, taking medications, or have existing health conditions.

Artichoke Leaf

Artichoke leaf is well-known for its ability to support bile flow, making it easier for your liver to break down fats and flush out waste. It contains cynarin, a compound that helps protect liver cells and even supports their regeneration. Adding artichoke leaf to your routine is a great way to enhance digestion and promote overall liver health.

Things to Consider: This herb may not be suitable for individuals with gallstones or bile duct blockages. If you experience digestive discomfort or have gallbladder issues, check with your doctor before using it.

Chicory Root

Chicory root is a soothing herb that promotes liver detoxification by increasing bile production and helping your body eliminate waste more efficiently. It also acts as a prebiotic, feeding the good bacteria in your gut—an essential factor in maintaining both digestive and liver health. Sipping on chicory root tea is a simple and natural way to support your liver.

Things to Consider: Chicory root can sometimes cause bloating or gas if consumed in large quantities. It may also trigger allergic reactions in people sensitive to ragweed or related plants. Start with small amounts and consult a healthcare provider if you have allergies.

Dandelion Root

Dandelion root is a fantastic herb for supporting liver health. It encourages your liver to produce bile, which aids in digesting fats and removing toxins from the body. Packed with antioxidants, dandelion root also helps protect liver cells from damage caused by free radicals. Whether enjoyed as a tea or taken as a supplement, it's a gentle yet effective way to detox and boost liver function.

Things to Consider: Dandelion root may cause allergic reactions in people sensitive to plants like ragweed or daisies. It can also interact with medications like diuretics or blood thinners. If you're on medication or have allergies, consult your healthcare provider before use.

Licorice Root

Licorice root is a calming herb with impressive anti-inflammatory and antioxidant properties. It can help balance liver enzymes, reduce oxidative stress, and support the repair of liver tissue. This makes it especially beneficial for anyone experiencing liver inflammation or looking to protect their liver from damage.

Things to Consider: Licorice root can raise blood pressure and lower potassium levels, so it's not suitable for people with high blood pressure, kidney disease, or heart conditions. It may also interact with medications like corticosteroids or diuretics. Avoid long-term use and always consult a doctor before starting.

Schisandra Berry

Schisandra berry is an adaptogenic herb that works wonders for the liver. It helps the liver process toxins more efficiently while protecting it from damage caused by free radicals. Rich in antioxidants and lignans, schisandra also supports liver regeneration and boosts energy, making it a valuable addition to any liver health plan.

Things to Consider: This herb may not be suitable for people with epilepsy, GERD, or other gastrointestinal conditions due to its stimulating effects. It can also interact with medications metabolized by the liver. If you're taking medications or have existing conditions, consult your healthcare provider.

Milk Thistle

One of the most well-known herbs for liver health. It contains silymarin, a compound believed to reduce liver inflammation and promote the regeneration of liver cells. It's often used as a complementary therapy for liver conditions, though you should consult a healthcare professional before starting any supplement (Kubala, 2023).

Things to Consider: Milk thistle is generally safe but may cause mild digestive upset in some individuals. People allergic to ragweed or related plants should use it cautiously. If you're on medication that affects the liver, consult your doctor before use.

Turmeric

Turmeric is a golden spice celebrated for its anti-inflammatory and antioxidant properties. Curcumin, its active ingredient, helps reduce liver inflammation and supports detoxification by promoting bile production. Adding turmeric to your diet or taking it as a supplement can benefit liver health.

Things to Consider: Turmeric may not be suitable for individuals with gallbladder issues or those on blood-thinning medications. High doses can sometimes cause digestive upset. Always consult a healthcare provider for proper guidance on how much to take.

If you're looking for an antioxidant boost, try incorporating green tea or turmeric into your daily routine. You can sip on green tea in the afternoon or sprinkle turmeric into soups or stir-fries. Just remember to use supplements cautiously and consult a healthcare provider to ensure they're safe for you.

Practical Tips for Reducing Alcohol Intake and Quitting Smoking

Both alcohol consumption and smoking pose serious risks to liver health. Alcohol is processed by the liver, and chronic consumption can worsen liver inflammation. It, again, results in cirrhosis or liver failure. Smoking also introduces harmful toxins into the bloodstream, increasing the liver's workload and potentially worsening liver damage.

Reducing Alcohol Intake

While complete abstinence from alcohol is often recommended for those with liver disease, reducing intake can still have significant benefits if quitting altogether isn't an immediate option. Setting realistic goals and finding alternatives to alcohol in social settings can make this lifestyle change more manageable.

1. **Start Small:** Begin by cutting back on the number of drinks you have per week. If you typically have five, try reducing it to three, then two.
2. **Replace alcoholic drinks:** Swap out alcoholic beverages for healthier options, like sparkling water with lemon or non-alcoholic cocktails.
3. **Social strategies:** In social settings, explain to friends or family that you're cutting back on your health. Having supportive people around you can make it easier to stick to your goals.

Quitting smoking is another step in protecting your liver. Smoking contributes to oxidative stress and inflammation, both of which can accelerate liver damage. While quitting smoking is challenging, the benefits to liver health—and overall well-being—are undeniable.

Some natural remedies can help curb the cravings associated with quitting smoking, although they should always be used in conjunction with a structured quit plan.

- **Licorice root:** Used as a natural aid to reduce nicotine cravings, licorice root can lower the urge to smoke. It also has mild anti-inflammatory properties that can support liver health (Kubala, 2023).
- **Lobelia:** Known for its potential to reduce nicotine cravings, lobelia is an herb that some people use during their quitting journey. However, it should only be used under professional supervision due to its potency (Streit, 2024).

Let's meet John, a 45-year-old with fatty liver disease. He found it tough to quit drinking entirely but started by replacing his evening glass of wine with herbal tea. He also used licorice root supplements to help reduce his cravings for cigarettes, gradually weaning himself off both habits over time.

While herbal remedies can support liver health, it's important to approach them with caution. Some supplements are not regulated as strictly as medications, and in rare cases, they may even harm the liver, especially if taken in high doses or alongside other medications.

For example, *kava,* an herb sometimes used to relieve anxiety, has been linked to liver toxicity and should be avoided by anyone with liver disease (Kandola, 2018). Similarly, high doses of vitamin A can be harmful to the liver, so it's important to monitor supplement intake and avoid megadoses (Kubala, 2023a).

Maintaining a Healthy Liver for Life

Maintaining a healthy liver is a lifelong commitment, and it's one that pays off in countless ways. The liver plays a central role in almost every metabolic process, from detoxification to digestion, so keeping it in top shape is essential for overall well-being. The good news is that many of the lifestyle changes that promote liver health also improve your general health, energy levels, and even mood.

Let us explore practical and sustainable ways to maintain liver health for life, focusing on nutrition, exercise, hydration, stress management, and regular health check-ups.

Prioritize a Nutrient-Rich Diet

The foundation of liver health starts with what you eat. The liver processes everything that enters your body, so you need to fuel it with foods that support its functions and minimize those that strain it. A balanced diet that includes a variety of nutrient-dense foods can prevent liver diseases like non-alcoholic fatty liver disease (NAFLD) and keep your liver functioning efficiently.

As mentioned earlier, whole foods, such as vegetables, fruits, whole grains, lean proteins, and healthy fats are the building blocks of a liver-friendly diet. They provide the vitamins, minerals, and fiber your liver needs to perform its detoxifying functions while minimizing fat accumulation. To explore more about detoxification and overall health, you can also check out my other works, including *Why We Need to Detox* and *Detox Our Brain* in the *Things We Need To Do* series.

One of the biggest culprits in liver damage is excess sugar. High levels of fructose (found in sugary drinks and processed foods) can overload the liver, leading to fat buildup and inflammation. Processed foods, especially those high in trans fats and artificial additives, can also strain the liver's ability to detoxify the body.

Stay Physically Active

Exercise isn't just good for your heart and muscles; it's also a powerful tool for maintaining liver health. Regular physical activity can help prevent liver disease by promoting healthy weight management, improving insulin sensitivity, and reducing liver fat. Even moderate exercise can make a significant difference.

Water plays an often-overlooked role in liver health. It helps the liver process and eliminates toxins from the body, so staying well-hydrated ensures that your liver can do its job efficiently. Dehydration can cause toxins to build up, straining the liver and impairing its ability to metabolize nutrients and fats.

Why Hydration Matters

Your liver depends on adequate hydration to maintain optimal blood flow and flush out waste products. Drinking enough water also aids in digestion, helping the liver break down fats and sugars more effectively. Additionally, proper hydration supports kidney function, which works hand-in-hand with the liver to cleanse the body.

You can keep a water bottle with you throughout the day and aim to drink around 8 glasses of water daily. If you find plain water boring, try infusing it with slices of lemon, cucumber, or mint for a refreshing twist. Herbal teas can also contribute to your daily hydration goal.

Manage Stress for a Healthier Liver

Chronic stress can take a toll on your liver. When you're stressed, your body produces hormones like cortisol and adrenaline, which can lead to inflammation and increase the workload on your liver. Over time, unmanaged stress can contribute to liver diseases, as it often correlates with unhealthy behaviors such as poor diet, lack of sleep, and excessive alcohol consumption.

Mindfulness practices, such as meditation, yoga, and deep breathing exercises, are excellent ways to manage stress. These techniques not only calm your mind but also lower cortisol levels, which can reduce liver inflammation. Even just ten minutes of deep breathing or meditation each day can make a difference.

Regular Health Check-Ups and Liver Screenings

Routine health check-ups cannot be ignored for maintaining liver health, especially as you age or if you have risk factors such as obesity, diabetes, or a family history of liver disease. Regular screenings can detect early signs of liver dysfunction or disease, allowing for timely intervention.

Early detection is key to preventing liver disease progression. Blood tests that measure liver enzymes (like ALT and AST) can reveal early signs of liver inflammation, while imaging tests (such as ultrasounds or FibroScan) can assess liver fat levels or scarring. Your doctor may also recommend lifestyle changes based on these results to help protect your liver long-term.

Avoid Toxins and Chemicals

Your liver works hard to detoxify harmful substances from your body, but exposure to environmental toxins, chemicals, and pollutants can overburden it. Avoiding certain toxins, whether they come from cleaning products, personal care items, or even the air you breathe—can reduce your liver's workload and minimize the risk of liver damage.

Minimizing Toxin Exposure

Minimizing your toxin exposure is also important for maintaining good health and improving your overall well-being. One area where you can make significant changes is in your household products. Many traditional cleaning supplies contain harsh chemicals that can be harmful to both the environment and your body. Instead, you can opt for natural and non-toxic cleaning products. These products are often made from ingredients that are safe for you and your pets. For example, baking soda and vinegar can effectively clean surfaces and eliminate odors without exposing you to dangerous chemicals. When shopping, you should look for labels that indicate the product is environmentally friendly. This also helps you support brands that prioritize health and sustainability.

In the realm of personal care, you should pay attention to the ingredients found in your skincare and cosmetic products. Many widely used products contain harmful chemicals like parabens, phthalates, and sulfates, which can disrupt your hormonal balance and cause skin irritations. Choosing products that are free from these substances is a wise decision. Look for labels that highlight 'clean,' 'natural,' or 'organic' ingredients. A great way for you to start is by replacing one product at a time with a safer alternative. For instance, if you regularly use a moisturizer that lists several synthetic ingredients, consider switching to one made from natural oils, such as coconut or almond oil. These alternatives can be just as effective, if not more so, in maintaining your skin health.

Another critical aspect involves pollution, particularly air pollution, which can have significant negative effects on your overall health. To reduce your exposure to pollution, especially if you live in urban areas, it's wise for you to keep an eye on local air quality reports. On days when air pollution levels are high, you should avoid outdoor exercise. Instead, consider indoor workouts, which can include activities like yoga or strength training. If staying indoors isn't possible for you, try to limit the time you spend outside when pollution levels are elevated.

Indoors, using air purifiers can greatly enhance your air quality, making your environment safer and more pleasant. Air purifiers remove contaminants like dust, pet dander, and smoke particles from the air, helping you breathe easier. When choosing an air purifier, consider one with a true HEPA filter, as these are designed to trap tiny particles that can be harmful when inhaled. Placing air purifiers in the main areas of your home, like the living room and bedroom, contributes to a healthier living environment for you.

Additionally, it may be helpful for you to monitor other sources of toxins in your home. For instance, consider the materials used in your furnishings and building supplies. Opt for furniture made from natural wood rather than particleboard, which can emit harmful gases. When renovating, look for low-VOC (volatile organic compounds) paints and finishes. These products are less likely to release harmful chemicals into the air and help improve your indoor environment.

In the kitchen, be mindful of the cookware you use. Non-stick pans are convenient but can sometimes release toxic substances if heated too high. Instead, consider using stainless steel, cast iron, or ceramic cookware, which are safer options for your meals. These materials not only cook food evenly but also don't leach harmful substances into your meals.

In summary, minimizing your toxin exposure can be accomplished in various aspects of your life. By making informed choices about household products, personal care items, and your surrounding environment, you can significantly improve your health and wellness. Taking small, actionable steps like switching to natural cleaning supplies, opting for clean beauty products, monitoring air quality, and being cautious about indoor materials can make a big difference for you. Each of these changes contributes to a healthier lifestyle, one choice at a time.

Real-Life Success Stories

In a compelling case study, a 56-year-old woman faced the daunting diagnosis of non-alcoholic fatty liver disease (NAFLD) alongside diabetes and obesity. Weighing 220 pounds and having a body mass index (BMI) of 36, she was determined to reclaim her health. Driven to prevent further complications, she began a life-changing journey, embracing a complete overhaul of her lifestyle.

Her regimen focused on a low-calorie, low-carbohydrate diet enriched with protein and healthy fats, complemented by regular physical activity. She embraced activities like walking and swimming, gradually increasing her endurance. Additionally, she prioritized mental well-being through mindfulness practices and stress reduction techniques.

Within six months, her dedication paid off. She successfully lost 25 pounds and saw significant improvements in her liver enzymes, which indicated a reversal of NAFLD. This remarkable transformation not only enhanced her physical health but also boosted her confidence and overall quality of life.

This story underscores the power of commitment and the effectiveness of lifestyle changes in managing and reversing fatty liver disease. It serves as a reminder that with determination and the right approach, individuals can reclaim their health and vitality (Nong et al., 2022).

In another revealing case study, a 61-year-old man with non-alcoholic fatty liver disease (NAFLD) struggled with obesity and high blood pressure. Weighing 200 pounds with a BMI of 31, he faced serious health risks. After realizing the urgency of his situation, he committed to lifestyle changes that could turn things around.

He adopted a Mediterranean diet rich in fruits, vegetables, whole grains, and healthy fats while cutting back on sugars and processed foods. Alongside dietary changes, he engaged in regular exercise, focusing on both cardiovascular workouts and strength training.

Over the course of a year, his efforts paid off significantly. He lost 30 pounds and improved his liver function tests, leading to a remarkable reduction in liver fat. This transformation not only enhanced his physical health but also revitalized his outlook on life, demonstrating that with dedication and the right approach, individuals can effectively manage and reverse NAFLD (Oh et al., 2023).

Adapting to life with fatty liver disease involves practical changes and natural remedies that can support your liver health. Every small step contributes to your overall well-being.

Activity: Self-Care Plan Development: My Personalized Wellness Roadmap

Step 1: Reflect on Your Current Routine

1. Take a moment to observe your current daily routine. Write down your typical activities, from morning to night.
2. Identify areas of improvement by asking questions, like, "What habits make me feel good?" and "What could I change to feel even better?"

Step 2: Set Your Wellness Goals

1. Define your goals in specific areas, such as hydration, nutrition, exercise, and mindfulness.
2. Use SMART criteria to ensure your goals are Specific, Measurable, Achievable, Relevant, and Time-bound. For example: "I will drink nine glasses of water daily for the next month."

Step 3: Choose Positive Lifestyle Habits to Adopt

1. Pick a few habits you want to incorporate into your daily routine, like starting your day with a glass of water, practicing mindfulness for five minutes, or including more vegetables in your meals.
2. Make a list of these habits and decide how they fit into your current lifestyle.

Step 4: Create a Daily Routine Outline

1. Break down your day into morning, afternoon, and evening segments.

2. Assign specific actions for each part of the day to reinforce your wellness goals, such as a hydration goal in the morning or a relaxation routine before bed.

Step 5: Set a Timeline for Your Wellness Goals

1. Create realistic timelines for each goal. For example, you can aim to achieve a full hydration goal in two weeks or integrate daily mindfulness within one month.
2. Track your progress regularly to see how you're doing and adjust timelines if necessary.

Step 6: Identify Mindful Moments for Stress Reduction

1. Pinpoint moments in your day when you can practice mindfulness.
2. Incorporate simple mindfulness exercises, such as deep breathing, grounding techniques, or reflecting on what you're grateful for.

Step 7: Use the Wellness Roadmap Worksheet to Monitor Progress

1. Record your progress daily using a worksheet or journal. This will include checking off completed tasks, jotting down thoughts, and noting any challenges.
2. Celebrate small wins to stay motivated, and review your goals periodically to ensure they're still aligned with your needs.

11

Stay Ahead with Regular Check-ups

When it comes to our health, prevention is always better than cure, and regular check-ups are the key to catching potential problems before they become serious. This is especially true for those with liver disease, where symptoms often develop quietly, sometimes without any noticeable signs, until the condition has progressed. Regular check-ups become a vital tool in managing liver health, allowing you to stay on top of your progress and make adjustments to treatment plans as needed.

In this chapter, we'll dive into why regular medical monitoring is essential and how it can make all the difference in your long-term liver health.

The Importance of Monitoring Your Liver Health

We know that the liver is a resilient organ, capable of regenerating itself, but it can also suffer severe damage over time without noticeable symptoms. Many people live with liver disease for years before realizing it, which is why you need to have routine check-ups and tests

Liver Function Tests: What They Tell You

Routine liver function tests (LFTs) are a key part of liver health monitoring. These blood tests measure levels of liver enzymes, proteins, and bilirubin, all of which help evaluate how well the liver is performing its essential functions. Here are some common components of LFTs:

- **Alanine transaminase (ALT):** An enzyme found in the liver that helps metabolize proteins. High levels of ALT in the blood may indicate liver damage or inflammation.
- **Aspartate transaminase (AST):** Another enzyme that helps metabolize amino acids. Elevated AST levels can also signal liver injury.
- **Alkaline phosphatase (ALP):** This enzyme is involved in bile production. High levels can indicate blockages in the bile ducts or liver damage.
- **Bilirubin:** This is a waste product produced when red blood cells break down. Elevated bilirubin levels can indicate problems with liver function or bile flow.

These tests offer doctors a snapshot of how well the liver is functioning and can help detect issues, like liver inflammation, damage, or blockages. For those managing liver conditions like NAFLD (non-alcoholic fatty liver disease) or hepatitis, regular LFTs are very important for tracking the progress of the disease and ensuring that treatments are working.

One of the biggest advantages of regular liver monitoring is early detection. Conditions like fatty liver disease, hepatitis, and cirrhosis can all progress without noticeable symptoms, making regular check-ups essential for catching problems in their early stages. With early detection, treatment options are often less invasive and more effective.

If you are already managing liver disease, regular monitoring is important to ensure treatments are working. Whether you're taking medications to control inflammation, following a specific diet to reduce liver fat, or making lifestyle changes to improve liver function, check-ups provide vital feedback on how well those interventions are working.

One of the most important things to remember about liver health is that consistency matters. Regular monitoring isn't just about one-time testing; it's about establishing a routine of check-ups to ensure long-term health. For those at risk of liver disease or already managing it, regular check-ups provide peace of mind and allow for timely interventions.

Tips for Making the Most of Doctor Visits

Navigating healthcare visits can often feel hectic, especially when it involves managing a condition, like fatty liver disease or other liver-related health issues. Between understanding medical terminology, dealing with complex treatment plans, and ensuring you get the most out of your consultations, it's easy to feel lost. However, with a little preparation and understanding, you can make your healthcare visits more effective and less stressful. This section will provide you with practical tips for preparing for your appointments, communicating effectively with your healthcare providers, and making the most of your time in the clinic.

Preparing for Your Appointment

Preparation is the key to a successful healthcare visit. Taking the time to organize your thoughts, questions, and relevant health information can make your experience much smoother.

1. **Keep a health journal:** Start by maintaining a health journal where you can log symptoms, medications, dietary habits, and any changes you notice in your condition. This journal can serve as a valuable reference during your appointments, helping you recall important details that might affect your treatment plan. For example, if you've been experiencing fatigue or abdominal discomfort, note when these symptoms occur and any potential triggers (like certain foods or activities). When you share this information with your doctor, it can help them make more informed decisions about your care.
2. **List your medications:** Compile a list of all medications, supplements, and over-the-counter products you are currently taking. Include dosages and frequency. This information is critical, as it helps your doctor understand potential interactions or side effects that could impact your liver health. For example, if you take herbal supplements, like milk thistle or dandelion root, be sure to mention these to your healthcare provider. They can evaluate their effectiveness and whether they might interfere with other treatments.
3. **Prepare questions:** Write down any questions or concerns you have regarding your liver health or treatment options. Having these questions in front of you during the visit ensures you don't forget to address them, helping you gain a clearer understanding of your condition. You can ask:
    - What do my recent liver function tests indicate about my health?
    - Are there specific dietary changes I should implement?
    - How often should I schedule follow-up appointments?

- What signs should I watch for that might indicate my condition is worsening?

4. **Bring support:** If possible, bring a family member or friend to your appointment. Having someone else there can provide emotional support, help you remember the information discussed, and assist in asking questions you might forget. For instance, your companion can think of a question that you didn't consider, or they can help take notes during your appointment, allowing you to focus on the conversation.

Communicating Effectively with Your Healthcare Provider

Once you're in the appointment, effective communication is essential. Here are some tips to ensure you and your doctor are on the same page:

1. **Be honest and open:** Share all relevant information about your health, lifestyle, and any symptoms you're experiencing, no matter how minor they seem. This transparency allows your doctor to understand your situation better and tailor their advice accordingly. If you've been consuming more alcohol than recommended, let your doctor know.
2. **Ask for clarification:** If your doctor uses medical jargon or you don't understand something they say, don't hesitate to ask for clarification. It's essential that you fully comprehend your condition and treatment plan. If your doctor, for instance, mentions "transaminitis" and you're unsure what it means, ask them to explain it in simpler terms. Understanding your liver's condition is crucial for managing your health effectively.

3. **Summarize key points:** At the end of the appointment, summarize the key points discussed and any action items you need to follow. This practice helps ensure that you and your healthcare provider are aligned on the next steps. You can say, "So, to summarize, I'll continue taking my current medications, adjust my diet to include more whole foods, and schedule a follow-up in three months. Is that correct?" This confirms understanding and allows for any necessary adjustments.
4. **Take notes:** During the appointment, jot down important information, recommendations, and any changes to your treatment plan. Writing things down helps reinforce what you learned and serves as a reference for later. Note any dietary suggestions your doctor provides, such as specific foods to avoid or incorporate into your meals, so you can review them later.

Making the Most of Your Time in the Clinic

Time is often limited during medical appointments, so maximize the value of each visit. Here are some strategies to ensure you leave the clinic feeling informed and empowered:

1. **Prioritize your concerns**
2. **Request follow-up care**
3. **Utilize online resources**
4. **Stay engaged**

Handling Difficult Conversations

Sometimes, healthcare visits can lead to difficult conversations, especially when discussing diagnoses, treatment failures, or lifestyle changes. Here are some tips for navigating these challenging discussions:

1. **Prepare emotionally:** Before your appointment, mentally prepare yourself for potentially tough conversations. Recognize that discussing liver health may bring up anxiety, fear, or uncertainty, and that's okay. Acknowledging these feelings can help you approach the conversation with clarity. The sooner you discuss it with your doctor, the sooner you can take steps to manage your health.
2. **Practice empathy:** Remember that medical providers are there to help you. If you feel overwhelmed, don't hesitate to express your feelings to your doctor. A good healthcare provider will understand your concerns and work to address them compassionately. You can say, "I'm feeling really anxious about a possible cirrhosis diagnosis. Can we talk about what that would mean for my treatment options?" This openness fosters a supportive environment for discussing your concerns.
3. **Focus on solutions:** While it's important to address challenges, try to shift the conversation towards solutions and action steps. This proactive approach empowers you to take control of your health. If your doctor discusses the need for weight loss to improve your liver health, instead of feeling discouraged, ask, "What specific steps can I take to achieve this? Are there resources or programs you recommend?"
4. **Seek support:** If a conversation feels particularly daunting, consider bringing a trusted friend or family member to the appointment. They can provide emotional support and help you articulate your concerns. For instance, if you're discussing difficult

lifestyle changes, your support person can help remind you of your goals and provide encouragement throughout the conversation.

Post-Appointment Reflections

After your healthcare visit, take a few moments to reflect on the information you received and how it affects your liver health. Here are some practices to incorporate:

1. Go over the notes you took during the appointment and clarify any points that may be unclear. This review reinforces your understanding and prepares you for any next steps.
2. Based on your discussion, set specific, achievable goals for yourself. Whether it's adopting a new dietary approach, scheduling follow-up appointments, or starting a new exercise routine, clear goals keep you focused. If your doctor recommended cutting back on sugar, set a goal of reducing sugary snacks and beverages for the next month. Tracking your progress can help you stay accountable.
3. If you have any questions or concerns after your visit, don't hesitate to reach out to your healthcare provider. Sending a message through a patient portal or calling the office is perfectly acceptable.
4. Remember that managing your liver health is an ongoing journey. Stay proactive about monitoring your health, and don't hesitate to reach out to your healthcare team whenever you have concerns or need support.

Staying Proactive with Preventative Care

When it comes to managing liver health, staying proactive with preventative measures is key. It's not just about treating existing issues but also about adopting a lifestyle that minimizes the risk of further complications and enhances overall well-being.

This section will explore effective strategies for preventing liver disease, emphasizing the importance of regular check-ups, lifestyle modifications, and the power of education.

Understanding the Importance of Prevention

Preventative measures can help you take care of your liver health because they can help catch potential problems early, preventing them from escalating into serious conditions. One of the most impactful preventative measures for liver health is adopting a balanced diet, as discussed in the last chapters.

Staying proactive about liver health also involves more than just lifestyle changes; it also includes regular health screenings and check-ups with your healthcare provider.

1. **Routine blood tests:** Regular blood tests can help monitor liver function and detect any abnormalities. If you have a history of elevated liver enzymes, your doctor may recommend more frequent monitoring to ensure your liver remains healthy.
2. **Ultrasounds and imaging:** Depending on your risk factors and family history, your healthcare provider may recommend imaging tests, such as ultrasounds or MRIs, to assess liver size and detect any fatty deposits or other abnormalities.
3. **Vaccinations:** Stay up-to-date on vaccinations that protect against liver infections, such as hepatitis

A and B. These vaccinations are crucial, especially for those at higher risk of liver disease. For instance, if you travel frequently or work in healthcare, ensure you are vaccinated against hepatitis A and B, as exposure risks may be higher in these scenarios.

4. **Monitoring metabolic health**: Conditions like obesity, diabetes, and high blood pressure can increase the risk of fatty liver disease. Regular screenings for these conditions and managing them effectively are essential for liver health. If you have prediabetes, working with a dietitian to create a meal plan that focuses on low-GI foods and regular exercise can help improve insulin sensitivity and reduce the risk of fatty liver.

Creating a Supportive Environment

1. Surround yourself with a supportive network of family, friends, and healthcare providers. Share your health goals with them and let them know how they can assist you in maintaining a healthy lifestyle.
2. Regular communication with your healthcare team is essential. Don't hesitate to reach out to them with questions or concerns about your liver health or treatment plan.
3. Look for local or online support groups for people with fatty liver disease. Sharing experiences with others facing similar challenges can provide emotional support and valuable insights into managing your condition.

Activity: Liver Health Check-Up Challenge

This exercise will help you reflect on your current liver health practices, identify areas for improvement, and create a personalized action plan for better liver health.

Instructions: Follow the steps below and take a few moments to complete the challenge.

Step 1: Self-Assessment Quiz

Answer the following questions to gauge your current habits related to liver health:

1. **Do you have regular check-ups with your healthcare provider?**
   - Yes, I have them every 6 months.
   - Yes, once a year.
   - No, but I plan to start.
   - No, I don't see a need.
2. **How often do you consume alcohol?**
   - Never
   - Occasionally (one to two times a month)
   - Regularly (a few times a week)
   - Daily
3. **Do you maintain a balanced diet rich in fruits, vegetables, and whole grains?**
   - Always
   - Most of the time
   - Sometimes
   - Rarely
4. **Are you physically active?**
   - Yes, I exercise regularly (at least 3 times a week)
   - I try to be active but need improvement
   - I rarely exercise
   - No, I am inactive
5. **Do you track your medications and supplements?**

  - Yes, I keep a detailed log
  - I keep a mental note
  - No, but I plan to start
  - No, I don't see it as necessary

Step 2: Reflection

Based on your answers, reflect on the following:

- What areas are you doing well in?
- Which areas could use improvement?
- Are there specific changes you can make to enhance your liver health?

Step 3: Create Your Action Plan

Using your reflections, create a personalized action plan. Here's a template to help you:

1. **Goal:** (e.g., Increase vegetable intake; you can also use the meal plan discussed in chapter four)
   - **Action Steps:**
     - Try one new vegetable recipe each week.
     - Set a reminder to include vegetables in every meal.
2. **Goal:** (e.g., Schedule regular check-ups)
   - **Action Steps:**
     - Mark my calendar to schedule an appointment every six months.
     - Prepare a list of questions to ask during my next visit.
3. **Goal:** (e.g., Reduce alcohol consumption)
   - **Action Steps:**
     - Limit alcohol to special occasions.

- Replace alcoholic beverages with sparkling water or herbal tea.

Step 4: Share and Engage

Consider sharing your goals and action plan with a friend or family member who can support you in your journey toward better liver health. You could even create a small accountability group where everyone can share their progress and motivate each other!

12

The Power of Knowledge

Knowledge is your superpower. In an age where information is at our fingertips, education has become an invaluable tool in managing health conditions, particularly something as complex as fatty liver disease. Knowledge not only equips you with an understanding of your health but also empowers you to take charge of your well-being. Just as one would seek to understand the nuances of a new job or hobby, delving into the intricacies of liver health can lead to better decision-making, improved health outcomes, and a proactive approach to care.

This chapter will guide you through the plethora of resources available for further learning about fatty liver disease and overall liver health, making education an integral part of your journey.

Why Education is Key to Wellness

Education about health is not just about learning medical jargon or understanding disease processes; it's about gaining the confidence to advocate for oneself and to make informed choices that can positively impact one's quality of life. You will need to understand the condition, its causes, symptoms, treatment options, and lifestyle implications, as they can lead to better management strategies and the potential for reversal of the disease.

Being informed helps demystify medical processes, fosters open communication with healthcare providers, and creates a supportive environment for discussions about health. This proactive stance can make navigating the complexities of healthcare less daunting and more empowering.

Online Tools

1. **Reputable health websites:** There are numerous online platforms dedicated to educating the public about liver health. Websites such as the *American Liver Foundation* and the *National Institute of Diabetes and Digestive and Kidney Diseases (NIDDK)* offer comprehensive information about fatty liver disease, treatment options, and lifestyle changes that can enhance liver health. For example, by exploring these websites, you can access downloadable brochures, interactive tools, and links to support groups that further enrich your understanding of liver health.
   - **American Liver Foundation:** This site features a wealth of resources, including articles on various liver diseases, tips for healthy living, and information on clinical trials and research initiatives. Their patient education resources present clear explanations of conditions, like fatty liver disease, making complex information accessible.
   - **NIDDK:** This government resource offers an extensive overview of liver function, disease, and

management strategies. Their patient guides and research updates ensure that you receive accurate and up-to-date information.

2. **Online courses and webinars:** Many organizations offer free or low-cost online courses and webinars focused on liver health. These interactive sessions can cover a range of topics, from nutrition and exercise to managing liver disease. For example, a course on nutrition may help you understand how your dietary choices directly impact your liver health, equipping you with practical strategies for making healthier food selections.
   - **Coursera and edX:** Platforms like these often host courses created by universities or healthcare institutions that dive deep into subjects related to health and wellness. Topics may include nutrition science, metabolic health, and the role of the liver in overall bodily function.
3. **YouTube channels:** Various healthcare professionals and organizations maintain educational YouTube channels that focus on liver health. These channels often provide insights through engaging videos that explain complex concepts in easy-to-understand formats.
   - The *American Liver Foundation* and *Medscape* have channels that give educational content ranging from basic liver anatomy to specific discussions about liver diseases. Watching videos can be an effective way for visual learners to grasp important concepts.
4. **Social media and blogs:** Following healthcare professionals, nutritionists, and patient advocacy organizations on social media can help you stay in touch with continuous education and updates. Many of these platforms share personal stories, tips, and

resources that can empower your living with liver disease. Reading about someone's journey with fatty liver disease can offer you hope and practical strategies when facing similar circumstances. A blog post detailing dietary changes that led to improved liver health can inspire you to adopt similar practices.

- **Health blogs:** Blogs by registered dietitians or liver specialists often feature personal experiences and practical advice for managing fatty liver disease. They can provide relatable content, highlighting everyday challenges and solutions.

Books and Publications

1. **Health books:** Numerous books are available that focus on liver health and fatty liver disease, providing in-depth information, personal stories, and practical advice.
2. **Research articles and journals:** For those interested in the scientific aspects of fatty liver disease, academic journals, and research articles can provide valuable insights into the latest findings and treatment strategies. A research article, for example, on the efficacy of certain dietary patterns in reversing fatty liver disease can help inform your dietary choices and motivate discussions with healthcare providers.
   - **Journal success:** Websites like *PubMed* and *Google Scholar* allow you to search for articles and studies related to liver health. Reading peer-reviewed research can help individuals understand the current landscape of liver disease management.
3. **Support group materials:** Many support groups provide educational resources tailored to

those affected by fatty liver disease. These materials often cover emotional well-being, dietary tips, and success stories. For example, joining a support group can help you understand educational materials and gain a sense of community. This platform will help everyone learn from each other's journeys and support one another through challenges.

- **Local support groups:** Organizations like the American Liver Foundation often host local support groups where members can share experiences and learn from one another. Many of these groups also offer printed materials or access to online resources.

Last but not least, one of the most reliable sources of information about liver health is a healthcare professional. Specialists, such as hepatologists, dietitians, and primary care physicians, can give personalized guidance and educational materials tailored to individual needs.

Community Groups

1. **Local health departments:** Many local health departments offer resources and education on liver health, often through community workshops, health fairs, and educational seminars. For example, attending a local health fair may give you access to screenings, educational materials, and expert speakers who can provide insights into liver health.
    - **Engaging the community:** Participating in local health events can provide valuable information while also connecting you with others in your area who are interested in improving their health.

2. **Nonprofit organizations:** Nonprofit organizations focused on liver health often provide educational resources, support groups, and advocacy initiatives. Engaging with these organizations can provide valuable knowledge and support. Organizations like the *American Association for the Study of Liver Diseases (AASLD)* offer educational materials and updates on research advancements. Engaging with these organizations can provide valuable insights into the latest developments in liver disease management.

Becoming a Liver Health Advocate

By becoming an advocate for liver health, you can improve not only your own health outcomes but also raise awareness and support others facing similar challenges.

This subtopic will explore what it means to be an advocate, how to get involved, and the positive impact advocacy can have on both personal and community levels.

Understanding Advocacy

Advocacy encompasses taking action to support a cause or a group of people. In the context of liver health, it means promoting awareness, understanding, and effective management of liver diseases. This can take many forms, from educating yourself and others about liver health to participating in campaigns that aim to improve health policies and resources for liver disease patients.

Why Advocacy Matters

1. **Raising awareness:** One of the most significant roles of advocacy is to raise awareness about liver

health issues. Many people may not know about fatty liver disease or its potential complications. By sharing information, statistics, and personal stories, advocates can shine a light on the condition, helping to educate the public. For example, you can host an informational seminar or write articles for community newsletters that can help spread the word about the risks of fatty liver disease, its causes, and the importance of early detection.

2. **Supporting research and funding:** Advocacy can lead to increased funding for research into liver diseases, which can ultimately improve treatment options and patient care. Engaging with organizations that focus on liver health can amplify efforts to secure funding for research initiatives. For instance, you can join or support groups like the *American Liver Foundation*, which actively seeks donations and partnerships to fund research projects. Plus, they can have a direct impact on the advancement of liver disease treatments.
3. **Influencing policy changes:** Advocacy efforts can help influence healthcare policies that affect liver disease patients. By voicing concerns to lawmakers and participating in campaigns that promote better healthcare access and affordability, you can drive change at the legislative level. Participating in rallies or writing to representatives about the need for more comprehensive healthcare coverage for liver disease treatments can push policymakers to take action.

To become an advocate for liver health, start by educating yourself about liver conditions and treatments through books, seminars, and reputable online resources. Share your personal experiences to connect with others and engage with advocacy organizations to amplify your efforts. Utilize social media to spread awareness, promote preventative measures, and foster a supportive community around liver health issues.

Encouraging Others in Their Journey

Encouragement can be a powerful motivator for you if you are dealing with the challenges of a chronic illness. It provides emotional support, reinforces positive behaviors, and helps you feel less isolated. Encouragement is especially helpful in health journeys, where you may encounter setbacks, doubts, and frustration. A simple word of kindness or a supportive gesture can inspire hope and resilience.

Consider a person who has recently been diagnosed with fatty liver disease. They may feel overwhelmed by the lifestyle changes they need to make. A friend who checks in regularly, shares resources, or simply listens can help them feel understood and motivated to take action.

Practical Ways to Encourage Others

1. **Listen actively:**

One of the most effective ways to encourage someone is to listen actively. Sometimes, others just need a space to express their thoughts and feelings without judgment. By being present and listening, you show that you care and validate their experiences.

- Set aside time for conversations.
- Ask open-ended questions about their feelings and experiences.
- Resist the urge to jump in with advice unless they ask for it.
- Your attentive listening can be incredibly reassuring.

. . .

2. **Share information and resources:**

PROVIDING helpful information and resources can empower you to take charge of your health. This may include sharing articles, websites, or local resources related to fatty liver disease and healthy living. For example, if someone is struggling with dietary changes, share recipes or meal plans that are liver-friendly. You can also recommend apps that help track food intake or physical activity, making it easier for them to stay on track.

3. **Set goals together:**

Encouraging someone to set realistic, achievable goals can help them stay motivated. Working together to establish these goals not only makes them feel supported but also builds accountability.

- Sit down with them to discuss their health objectives, whether it's losing weight, exercising more, or reducing alcohol intake.
- Help them break these goals into smaller and manageable steps.
- Celebrate each small victory along the way, reinforcing their progress.

4. **Engage in healthy activities together:**

Sometimes, the best encouragement comes from shared experiences. Engaging in healthy activities together not only promotes good habits but also strengthens your bond. For example, you can Invite your friend to join you for a healthy cooking class or a fitness class. You can also schedule regular walks or hikes to promote physical activity and offer a supportive environment to talk about your health journey.

5. **Be a source of positive reinforcement:**

Positive reinforcement can be a powerful motivator. Celebrate their achievements, no matter how small, and remind them of their progress. Acknowledging their hard work can help them feel more confident in their journey. You can send a thoughtful message after they accomplish a goal, such as completing a week of healthy meals or attending a support group. Remind them of the importance of their journey and how far they've come.

6. **Create a supportive environment:**

Encouragement thrives in a supportive environment. Whether it's organizing group activities or forming a support group, creating a space where people can share their challenges and triumphs fosters camaraderie and motivation.

- Start a local support group for people dealing with fatty liver disease.
- This can be a safe space for sharing experiences, providing tips, and encouraging each other.
- Facilitating discussions about challenges and successes can help everyone feel less isolated.

7. **Lead by example:**

Your actions can inspire others more than words alone. Demonstrating a commitment to your own health and wellness can motivate those around you to take their health seriously.

- Share your own journey, whether you're making dietary changes, exercising more, or managing stress.
- By showing your dedication to healthy living, you can encourage others to follow suit.

8. **Encourage professional help:**

Sometimes, encouragement may also mean guiding others to seek professional help. Whether it's a nutritionist, therapist, or medical professional, the right guidance can lead to significant improvements in their health journey.

- Help them find reputable healthcare providers who specialize in liver health.
- Encourage them to attend counseling or therapy if they are struggling emotionally, as mental well-being is crucial for overall health.

9. **Stay connected:**

Regular check-ins can show that you care about their progress. Consistently reaching out can remind them that they're not alone in their journey.

- Set reminders to reach out, whether through texts, calls, or in-person visits.
- Ask them how they're doing and be prepared to listen and offer support as needed.

By leveraging reputable online resources, engaging with community organizations, and consulting healthcare professionals, you can empower them with the knowledge to advocate for their well-being.

Exercise 1: Resource Exploration Challenge

Objective: Familiarize yourself with credible resources about fatty liver disease.

1. **Choose two resources:** Select two different types of resources from the list provided (e.g., a website and a YouTube channel, or a health book and a blog).
2. **Explore:** Spend at least 30 minutes exploring each resource. Take notes on key takeaways, new information, or questions that arise.
3. **Reflect:** Write a short paragraph on how this new information can impact your understanding or management of fatty liver disease. Consider sharing your insights with a friend or in a support group.

Exercise 2: Advocacy Action Plan

Objective: Take steps toward becoming an advocate for liver health.

1. **Choose your focus:** Identify one area of liver health advocacy that resonates with you, such as raising awareness, supporting research, or influencing policy.
2. **Action steps:** Create a list of three concrete actions you can take to advocate for this cause. For example, you may decide to write an article for your community newsletter, organize a local health workshop, or join a liver health organization.
3. **Implementation:** Set a timeline for when you will complete each action step. Share your plan with someone who can support you in your advocacy efforts.

Conclusion

As we draw this journey to a close, let's reflect on the key strategies and messages that have emerged throughout the book regarding the management and potential reversal of fatty liver disease. Managing this chronic condition can feel difficult, but with the right knowledge, tools, and support, you can take significant steps toward improving your liver health and overall well-being.

At the heart of managing fatty liver disease is a holistic approach that emphasizes the interconnectedness of various lifestyle factors. Diet, exercise, mental health, and regular medical check-ups form the pillars of a comprehensive strategy aimed at tackling this condition. Each element plays a crucial role, and together, they create a supportive framework that fosters recovery and resilience.

Throughout our discussions, we've highlighted the pivotal role of diet in managing fatty liver disease. By focusing on whole foods, such as fruits, vegetables, lean proteins, and healthy fats, you can provide your liver with the nutrients it needs to function optimally. Foods that are low on the glycemic index help maintain stable blood sugar levels, which is vital for preventing further liver fat accumulation.

Imagine replacing processed snacks with fresh fruit or swapping sugary beverages for herbal teas. These small dietary changes can have a profound impact on your liver health. Incorporating antioxidants found in colorful fruits and vegetables can also help reduce inflammation and support liver function. For instance, including more blueberries, spinach, or nuts in your diet can boost your antioxidant intake, contributing positively to liver health.

Moreover, understanding the role of herbal supplements can complement dietary efforts. Supplements like milk thistle and turmeric have shown promise in supporting liver health. However, you need to consult with a healthcare professional before introducing any new supplements into your regimen.

Exercise is another cornerstone of managing fatty liver disease. Engaging in regular physical activity not only aids in weight management but also improves insulin sensitivity and promotes overall metabolic health. Even simple activities, such as walking, swimming, or cycling, can make a difference. Imagine incorporating a daily 30-minute walk into your routine, it can become a delightful way to unwind while supporting your liver.

The benefits of exercise extend beyond the physical. Engaging in group activities, such as yoga or dance classes, can also foster social connections, providing emotional support that is vital for mental health. Exercise acts as a natural stress reliever, helping to combat the anxiety and frustration that often accompany chronic health issues. As we discussed in earlier chapters, reducing stress through physical activity can have a direct positive effect on liver health, reinforcing the connection between mind and body.

Recognizing the importance of mental health in this journey is necessary. Chronic conditions can take a toll on emotional well-being, leading to feelings of isolation, frustration, or even depression. This is why adopting mindfulness practices and engaging in supportive communities can be transformative. Techniques like meditation and deep breathing exercises can help manage stress and cultivate a more positive mindset.

Consider the difference between approaching your health journey with a mindset focused on frustration versus one centered on empowerment. Seeking therapy or joining support groups can provide a safe space to share experiences and feelings. By encouraging open conversations about mental health, we can dismantle the stigma often associated with chronic illnesses and create an environment where healing can flourish.

Regular medical check-ups are an integral part of a successful health strategy. Monitoring your liver health through routine screenings and consultations with healthcare professionals allows for early detection of potential issues and timely interventions. As we've emphasized throughout this book, staying proactive in your healthcare is not merely about treatment; it's about empowerment.

Understanding your liver health status and collaborating with medical professionals enables you to make informed decisions about your care. For example, if blood tests indicate elevated liver enzymes, working with your doctor to adjust your lifestyle accordingly can help mitigate further damage. Remember, regular check-ups are not just a formality; they are an opportunity for you to advocate for your health and take charge of your journey.

Knowledge is power, and throughout this book, we've aimed to equip you with valuable information about fatty liver disease. By educating yourself, you gain the tools necessary to advocate for your health effectively. This empowerment extends beyond your personal journey; it can inspire those around you to take similar proactive steps.

As you become more informed, don't hesitate to share your knowledge with others. Whether it's discussing dietary changes with friends or encouraging family members to join you in healthy activities, your advocacy can create a ripple effect. Imagine leading by example, showing others how positive changes in lifestyle can improve overall well-being. Your journey can motivate someone else to take their health seriously, forging a community committed to better health.

Now that you are armed with insights about managing and reversing fatty liver disease, it's time to take action. Start with small, manageable steps—whether it's cooking a healthy meal, committing to regular exercise, or scheduling your next check-up. Each decision you make contributes to your journey of improving liver health.

Consider setting specific, achievable goals for yourself. Perhaps you aim to incorporate more fruits and vegetables into your meals, or maybe you commit to walking for 30 minutes a day. As you achieve these milestones, take a moment to celebrate your progress. Recognizing your accomplishments, no matter how small, fosters motivation and reinforces positive behaviors.

Living with fatty liver disease can be challenging, but it is also an opportunity for growth, resilience, and transformation. By embracing a holistic approach that prioritizes diet, exercise, mental health, and regular medical care, you can significantly improve your liver health and overall quality of life.

Remember, this journey is not meant to be walked alone. Seek support from healthcare professionals, friends, and community members who share your commitment to better health.

Together, we can create an environment that empowers individuals to thrive, advocating for themselves and each other in the pursuit of optimal liver health.

As you move forward, let the knowledge you've gained empower you to take control of your health. Each step you take—whether big or small—brings you closer to a healthier future. Embrace the journey ahead, armed with understanding, support, and the determination to live a vibrant, healthy life.

I truly hope this book has provided you with valuable insights and practical steps to improve your health. Your feedback means the world to me, and it helps others discover the book as well.

If you could take a moment to share your thoughts in a review, I'd be incredibly grateful. Visit your original order page or head to www.magletpublishing.com to leave your review. Your voice can make a difference!

Thank you so much for your support!

Other books you might enjoy by Sacha Lucas:

Things We Need To Do series

Detox Our Brain – 10 Strategies for Brain Health and Wellness
Why We Need To Detox – The Benefits of Detoxing Your Body to Reduce Gut Inflammation, Bloating, and Brain Fog

References

Arvind, A., Osganian, S. A., Cohen, D. E., & Corey, K. E. (2000). *Lipid and lipoprotein metabolism in liver disease* (K. R. Feingold, B. Anawalt, A. Boyce, G. Chrousos, K. Dungan, A. Grossman, J. M. Hershman, G. Kaltsas, C. Koch, P. Kopp, M. Korbonits, R. McLachlan, J. E. Morley, M. New, L. Perreault, J. Purnell, R. Rebar, F. Singer, D. L. Trence, & A. Vinik, Eds.). PubMed; MDText.com, Inc. https://www.ncbi.nlm.nih.gov/books/NBK326742/

Cherney, K. (2023, October 12). *6 liver-friendly foods to eat*. Healthline; Healthline Media. https://www.healthline.com/health/hepatitis-c/liver-friendly-foods-to-eat

Cleveland Clinic. (2021, November 4). *Alanine Transaminase (ALT) blood test: What it is, procedure & results*. Cleveland Clinic. https://my.clevelandclinic.org/health/diagnostics/22028-alanine-transaminase-alt

Collins, L., & Costello, R. A. (2023). *Glucagon-like peptide-1 receptor agonists*. PubMed; StatPearls Publishing. https://www.ncbi.nlm.nih.gov/books/NBK551568/

Cox, B., Trasolini, R., Galts, C., Yoshida, E. M., & Marquez, V. (2021). Comparing the performance of Fibrosis-4 and Non-Alcoholic Fatty Liver Disease Fibrosis Score with transient elastography scores of people with non-alcoholic fatty liver disease. *Canadian Liver Journal*, *4*(3), 275–282. https://doi.org/10.3138/canlivj-2021-0004

Coyle, D. (2023, February 24). *A beginner's guide to the low-glycemic diet*. Healthline. https://www.healthline.com/nutrition/low-glycemic-diet

Davis, C. P., & Memon, N. (2024, August 23). *Liver blood rests: AST normal range, results, function*. MedicineNet. https://www.medicinenet.com/liver_blood_tests/article.htm

Egan, M., & Prasad, S. (2011). Statins for patients with nonalcoholic fatty liver? *The Journal of Family Practice*, *60*(9), 536–538. https://www.ncbi.nlm.nih.gov/pmc/articles/PMC3183966/

Fletcher, J. (2022, July 15). *What to know about liver biopsy results*. Medical News Today. https://www.medicalnewstoday.com/articles/liver-biopsy-results

Fletcher, J., & Sissons, B. (2023, November 23). *AST (SGOT) blood test: High and low levels, and what do results mean*. Medical News Today. https://www.medicalnewstoday.com/articles/320982#faq

Foucher, J. (2006). Diagnosis of cirrhosis by transient elastography (FibroScan): a prospective study. *Gut*, *55*(3), 403–408. https://doi.org/10.1136/gut.2005.069153

Fowler, P. (2009, July 14). *Fatty liver: Causes, symptoms, and treatment*. WebMD; WebMD. https://www.webmd.com/hepatitis/fatty-liver-disease

Hashem, A., Khalouf, A., & Acosta, A. (2021). Management of obesity and nonalcoholic fatty liver disease: A literature review. *Seminars in Liver Disease*, *41*(4), 435–447. https://doi.org/10.1055/s-0041-1731704

Health direct. (2019, October 5). *Fatty liver*. Healthdirect; Healthdirect Australia. https://www.healthdirect.gov.au/fatty-liver

Huang, P. L. (2009). A comprehensive definition for metabolic syndrome. *Disease Models & Mechanisms*, *2*(5-6), 231–237. https://doi.org/10.1242/dmm.001180

Imai, K., Takai, K., Unome, S., Miwa, T., Hanai, T., Suetsugu, A., & Shimizu, M. (2023). FIB-4 index and NAFLD fibrosis score are useful indicators for screening high-risk groups of non-viral hepatocellular carcinoma. *Molecular and Clinical Oncology*, *19*(4). https://doi.org/10.3892/mco.2023.2676

Juo, Y.-Y., & Livingston, E. H. (2019, November 12). *Testing for nonalcoholic fatty liver disease*. JAMA. https://jamanetwork.com/journals/jama/fullarticle/2754794

Kandola, A. (2018, December 17). *Kava kava: Uses, benefits, risks, dosage, and interactions*. Medical News Today. https://www.medicalnewstoday.com/articles/324015

Knudsen, M. (2022, May 25). *Mediterranean diet for fatty liver: Does it help?* Healthline. https://www.healthline.com/nutrition/mediterranean-diet-for-fatty-liver

Kubala, J. (2023a, April 24). *Vitamin A: benefits, deficiency, toxicity and more*. Healthline; Healthline Media. https://www.healthline.com/nutrition/vitamin-a

Kubala, J. (2023b, September 12). *The 10 best herbs for liver health: Benefits and precautions*. Healthline. https://www.healthline.com/nutrition/herbs-for-liver

Kunnumakkara, A. B., Hegde, M., Kumar, A., Oommen, O. V., Aggarwal, B. B., Garodia, P., Yenisetti, S. C., Daimary, U. D., Girisa, S., & Parama, D. (2023). Role of turmeric and curcumin in prevention and treatment of chronic diseases: Lessons learned from clinical trials. *ACS Pharmacology & Translational Science*, *6*(4), 447–518. https://doi.org/10.1021/acsptsci.2c00012

Laursen, T. L., Hagemann, C. A., Wei, C., Kazankov, K., Thomsen, K. L., Knop, F. K., & Grønbæk, H. (2019). Bariatric surgery in patients with non-alcoholic fatty liver disease - from pathophysiology to clinical effects. *World Journal of Hepatology*, *11*(2), 138–149. https://doi.org/10.4254/wjh.v11.i2.138

Lefebvre, E., Moyle, G., Reshef, R., Richman, L. P., Thompson, M., Hong, F., Chou, Hsin-L., Hashiguchi, T., Plato, C., Poulin, D., Richards, T., Yoneyama, H., Jenkins, H., Wolfgang, G., & Friedman, S. L. (2016).

Antifibrotic effects of the dual CCR2/CCR5 antagonist cenicriviroc in animal models of liver and kidney fibrosis. *PloS One*, *11*(6), e0158156. https://doi.org/10.1371/journal.pone.0158156

Lian, J., & Fu, J. (2021). Pioglitazone for NAFLD patients with prediabetes or Type 2 diabetes mellitus: A meta-analysis. *Frontiers in Endocrinology*, *12*. https://doi.org/10.3389/fendo.2021.615409

McCommis, K. S., & Butler, A. A. (2020). The importance of keeping time in the liver. *Endocrinology*, *162*(2). https://doi.org/10.1210/endocr/bqaa230

Nevola, R., Imbriani, S., Tortorella, G., Aprea, C., Rinaldi, L., Epifani, R., Marfella, R., Sasso, F. C., & Galiero, R. (2023). *GLP-1 Receptor agonists in non-alcoholic fatty liver disease: Current evidence and future perspectives*. *24*(2), 1703–1703. https://doi.org/10.3390/ijms24021703

Newman, T. (2018, March 2). *The liver: structure, function, and disease*. Medical News Today. https://www.medicalnewstoday.com/articles/305075

Nong, Y.-B., Huang, H.-N., Huang, J.-J., Du, Y.-Q., Song, W.-X., Mao, D.-W., Zhong, Y.-X., Zhu, R.-H., Xiao, X.-Y., & Zhong, R.-X. (2022). Rare leptin in non-alcoholic fatty liver cirrhosis: A case report. *World Journal of Clinical Cases*, *10*(28), 10293–10300. https://doi.org/10.12998/wjcc.v10.i28.10293

Oh, Y. H., Jeong, S., Park, S. J., Ahn, J. C., & Park, S. M. (2023). Reversal of nonalcoholic fatty liver disease reduces the risk of cardiovascular disease among Korean. *Medicine*, *102*(44), e35804–e35804. https://doi.org/10.1097/md.0000000000035804

Rees, M. (2023, March 3). *What to know about vitamin E for fatty liver*. Medical News Today. https://www.medicalnewstoday.com/articles/vitamin-e-for-fatty-liver

Rich, N. E., Oji, S., Mufti, A. R., Browning, J. D., Parikh, N. D., Odewole, M., Mayo, H., & Singal, A. G. (2018). Racial and ethnic disparities in non-alcoholic fatty Liver disease prevalence, severity, and outcomes in the United States: A systematic review and meta-analysis. *Clinical Gastroenterology and Hepatology*, *16*(2), 198-210.e2. https://doi.org/10.1016/j.cgh.2017.09.041

Shah, R. A., & Kowdley, K. V. (2020). Obeticholic acid for the treatment of nonalcoholic steatohepatitis. *Expert Review of Gastroenterology & Hepatology*, *14*(5), 311–321. https://doi.org/10.1080/17474124.2020.1748498

Streit, L. (2024, September 26). *What Is lobelia, and how is it used?* Healthline; Healthline Media. https://www.healthline.com/nutrition/lobelia#benefits

Vere, C. C., Streba, C. T., Streba, L. M., Ionescu, A. G., & Sima, F. (2009). Psychosocial stress and liver disease status. *World Journal of Gastroenterology: WJG*, *15*(24), 2980–2986. https://doi.org/10.3748/wjg.15.2980

Wang, L., Cao, Z.-M., Zhang, L.-L., Li, J.-M., & Lv, W.-L. (2022). The role of gut microbiota in some liver diseases: From an immunological perspective.

Frontiers in Immunology, *13*, 923599. https://doi.org/10.3389/fimmu.2022.923599

Watson, S. (2024, January 26). *Ten foods to include in a healthy liver diet.* Healthline. https://www.healthline.com/health/fatty-liver-diet

WebMD Editorial Contributors. (2022, December 13). *What Is cortisol?* WebMD; WebMD. https://www.webmd.com/a-to-z-guides/what-is-cortisol

Xu, T., Li, L., Liu, Y., Cao, W., Chen, J., Hu, S., Liu, Y., Li, L., Zhou, H., Meng, X., Huang, C., Zhang, L., Li, J., & Zhou, H. (2020). CRISPR/Cas9-related technologies in liver diseases: from feasibility to future diversity. *International Journal of Biological Sciences*, *16*(13), 2283–2295. https://doi.org/10.7150/ijbs.33481

Yang, Z., & Wang, L. (2023). Current, emerging, and potential therapies for non-alcoholic steatohepatitis. *Frontiers in Pharmacology*, *14*. https://doi.org/10.3389/fphar.2023.1152042

Zhang, S., Mak, L.-Y., Yuen, M.-F., & Seto, W.-K. (2023). Screening strategy for non-alcoholic fatty liver disease. *Clinical and Molecular Hepatology*, *29*(Suppl), S103–S122. https://doi.org/10.3350/cmh.2022.0336

Author Bio

Sacha Lucas is an accomplished author, balancing a successful career, family life, and her own health journey. Diagnosed with an autoimmune disease at a young age, Sacha has spent decades learning to manage her physical and mental symptoms through trial, perseverance, and a deep commitment to natural healing. Her personal battle has led her to develop an expertise in detoxing the body and mind, which she now shares through her writing.

As the author of *Why We Need to Detox* and *Detox Our Brain* (both in the *Things We Need To Do* series), Sacha draws from both her personal experiences and extensive research to guide others on their own paths to wellness. In her latest book, *The Fatty Liver Fix*, she explores the critical importance of liver health, offering readers practical insights on reversing fatty liver disease through natural methods.

Sacha is dedicated to helping others discover their own strength and resilience, empowering them with the tools to detox their lives and achieve lasting health. With more books planned in the detox and wellness genre, Sacha is passionate about guiding her readers toward healthier, more vibrant living.

Made in United States
North Haven, CT
10 November 2026

22088339R00095